SIX RINGS

Signature Edition: Train the Mind, Rebuild the Body, Brain Wellness & Addiction Recovery: Before When Dragons Kill

Prof. Dr. Bankole Johnson, DSc., MD., MBChB., MPhil., DFAPA, DABDA, FACFEI, DAASCP

IRMN

Contents

Chapter 1
INTRODUCTION TO THE SIX RINGS

The Six Rings: Elemental Forces Within Us

There are frameworks that behave like filing cabinets: neat, labeled compartments that reassure the intellect but leave the soul untouched. And then there are frameworks that behave like maps: living instruments that help us orient when the terrain turns unfamiliar—when our minds race, our bodies rebel, our relationships fray, or the future feels heavier than we expected.

The Six Rings belong to the second kind.

To speak of "wellness" as if it were a single destination is one of our modern errors. Wellness is not a finish line; it is a *relationship*—a continuing negotiation between forces that shape us, within us and around us. Health is less like a static portrait and more like a symphony: countless parts, sometimes discordant, sometimes luminous, always in motion. We do not become well once and for all; we *practice* wellness the way we practice breathing, listening, adapting, and returning.

This is why the Six Rings can be understood not merely as "pillars" or "domains," but as elemental forces—fundamental modalities of nature that are also fundamental modalities of *being human*: **air, water, earth, sound, magnetism, and energy**. These are not poetic decorations laid over biology. They are biology's oldest metaphors—because they are biology's deepest realities.

Every person is an ecology. Every mind is a weather system. Every life is a field of influences. To pursue wellness is to learn how to read that field—how to recognize when one force is starved, when another is flooding, and how to restore balance without demanding perfection.

Because balance is not rigidity. Balance is *responsiveness*.

In the oldest philosophies, the elements were never merely "things." They were principles of movement, transformation, and order. In Greek thought, breath and spirit entwined as *pneuma*; in Hebrew, wind and spirit share a root in *ruach*; in Sanskrit, *prana* is both breath and life-force. Water is origin and return in myth and medicine. Earth is stability, nourishment, and consequence. Sound is creation, memory, and meaning. Magnetism is invisible influence—what pulls, what repels, what aligns. Energy is the currency of change, the possibility of action itself.

To bring these into one model is not to abandon science for poetry. It is to remember that the best science often begins where the best poetry lives: at the edge of what we can measure, in the place where experience becomes a question.

The Six Rings are the question made practical.

Air: The Ring of Breath, Space, and Choice

Air is the first rhythm of life, and the last. It is the most taken-for-granted medicine and the most underappreciated lever of change.

At the surface, air is oxygen—fuel for metabolism, the quiet partner of every cell that must convert nutrients into usable power. But air is also *space*: the capacity to pause, to widen the gap between stimulus and response, to create room where compulsion once lived.

This is not metaphor alone. The act of breathing is one of the rare bridges between the involuntary and the voluntary. You cannot simply *will* your heart rate into calm; but you can slow your exhale and watch your body follow. You can't argue your nervous system into safety; but you can train it, breath by breath, toward steadier ground.

In clinical language, breath is a gateway into autonomic regulation—into the balance between arousal and rest, vigilance and recovery. In human language, breath is the return of choice.

When air is out of balance, we see it everywhere:

- in shallow breathing that keeps the body braced,
- in the restless mind that cannot land,
- in the sense of being "crowded" from the inside,
- in craving, where urgency hijacks the future.

To restore the Air ring is to practice *presence as physiology*: not as a slogan, but as a lived ability to come back to the moment without being consumed by it. The breath becomes a teacher: steady, faithful, unimpressed by our stories, always offering another beginning.

Water: The Ring of Flow, Emotion, and Renewal

Water is the great mover. It travels. It carries. It dissolves. It cleans. It remembers.

Biologically, we are mostly water—not only in volume, but in function. Blood is a river. Lymph is a tide. Cerebrospinal fluid is a whispering current around the brain and spinal cord. Hydration affects circulation, temperature regulation, kidney function, cognition, and mood. But water is more than fluid balance. It is the body's language of *flow*.

Emotion itself is an ancient word: *e-motion*—energy in motion. When emotion is permitted to move, it becomes information. When emotion is dammed, it becomes pressure. When emotion is forced to vanish, it often returns as symptom—tightness, pain, insomnia, irritability, hunger that isn't hunger, thirst that isn't thirst.

In myth, water is cleansing because it restores continuity: it reconnects what has been fragmented. In psychology, water is the capacity to feel without drowning—to let experience pass through without becoming your identity.

When the Water ring is out of balance, we see:

- emotional rigidity (the inability to feel),
- emotional flooding (the inability to contain),
- bitterness that calcifies into worldview,
- the quiet dehydration of empathy—toward others and toward oneself.

Water asks for gentleness, but not weakness. It teaches that softness can be a strength: the strength to be honest, to grieve, to forgive, to let go, to begin again without denying what happened.

To restore Water is to restore *circulation*: in the body, yes—but also in the inner life. This is why so many healing traditions—ancient and modern—return to water in one form or another: bathing, immersion, tears, ritual washing, hydration, and the simple act of being near rivers, oceans, rainfall. We are not only healed by what we ingest, but by what we allow to move.

Earth: The Ring of Grounding, Structure, and Nourishment

Earth is the ring of *form*. The body is earth made animate: minerals shaped into bone, iron into blood, salts into electrical gradients, fats and proteins assembled into membranes and muscle. Even the word "human" whispers its kinship with soil —*humus*—as if language itself remembers that we are made of what we stand upon.

Earth is nutrition, yes—but also *structure*: sleep-wake rhythm, routine, boundaries, the built environment, the habits that hold us up when motivation fails. Earth is what makes healing durable.

In the modern world, we have an abundance of calories and a shortage of nourishment. We have endless stimulation and too little restoration. We have convenience and too little embodied wisdom. Earth reminds us that wellness cannot be sustained in abstraction. It must be built in the practical:

meals, movement, rest, sunlight, nature, community, and the daily actions that become the architecture of the self.

Earth is also our relationship with the living world: the microbiome that responds to what we eat and how we live; the way green spaces quiet stress responses; the way time outdoors recalibrates the sense of scale, returning us to something older than our anxieties.

When Earth is out of balance, we see:

- fragility where resilience should be,
- chaos disguised as freedom,
- impulsivity that feels like personality but is often physiology,
- a life that has no "floor" beneath it.

To restore Earth is to build a dependable baseline—the kind that makes excellence possible, not as perfection, but as steadiness. It is not glamorous. It is profoundly powerful.

Earth does not promise quick miracles. It promises something better: *capacity*.

Sound: The Ring of Resonance, Meaning, and Connection

Sound is the invisible architecture of experience. It enters us without asking permission. It shapes mood. It evokes memory. It organizes attention. It binds people together in time: lullabies, chants, hymns, national anthems, protest songs, love songs, the cadence of a trusted voice.

The ancients suspected that harmony governs reality—the "music of the spheres" in Pythagorean imagination, the idea that order can be heard as well as seen. Modern neuroscience, in its own language, echoes a cousin of that insight: rhythms matter. The brain is an organ of oscillations—patterns of synchronized activity that shift with sleep, learning, attention, and emotion. Even walking has a rhythm; conversation has a rhythm; relationships have a rhythm.

Sound, then, is not only what we hear. It is *how we attune*.

This is why music can steady anxiety, soften grief, and catalyze motivation. This is why rhythm can help movement disorders find their footing. This is why the tone of a room can change a nervous system before a single idea is spoken. Sound is a medicine because it is a form of patterned influence—resonance that reorganizes what has become scattered.

When Sound is out of balance, we see:

- a life filled with noise but starved of meaning,
- isolation that is not solved by company,
- a nervous system that cannot settle because it cannot "find the beat."

To restore Sound is to restore resonance: to choose what we listen to, to choose how we speak, to choose what we repeat in the mind as inner speech. It is also to rediscover awe—because awe is often the sound of the mind expanding.

In the beginning of many traditions, creation is described as sound: "the Word," the sacred syllable, the cosmic vibration. Whether taken literally or as metaphor, the wisdom stands: what we repeat shapes what we become.

Magnetism: The Ring of Alignment, Polarity, and Invisible Influence

Magnetism is the element most people treat as "mystical"

until they meet it in a scanner, a cardiac monitor, or a neuromodulation clinic. In truth, magnetism is simply a reminder of what has always been real: the most powerful forces are often invisible.

A human being is electrical. The heart is electrical. The brain is electrical. Nerves conduct signals through ionic gradients—tiny separations of charge that create the possibility of thought, movement, memory, and feeling. And wherever there is electricity, there is magnetism. The body is not only chemistry; it is also circuitry.

In medicine, magnetic modalities are no longer metaphor. Transcranial magnetic stimulation (TMS) uses magnetic fields to influence neural activity and has become a serious tool in neuropsychiatry. Imaging technologies reveal structure and function by leveraging magnetic principles. The "invisible influence" is measured, harnessed, and targeted.

But magnetism is also philosophical: it is the ring of *polarity*. We are pulled toward some things and repelled by others—habits, people, environments, substances, stories. Addiction itself can be described as pathological magnetism: a gravitational pull toward a short-term relief that steals the long-term future.

Magnetism asks a difficult and liberating question:

What is pulling you—and what are you practicing that makes you easier to pull?

When Magnetism is out of balance, we see:

- compulsions that feel fated,
- environments that "win" against good intentions,
- relationships that distort identity,

• relapse cycles where the same forces reassert themselves.

To restore Magnetism is to restore alignment. It is to change the field: cues, routines, supports, boundaries, treatments, and the deeper meaning that makes a person less susceptible to the tyranny of the immediate.

Magnetism is where modern science and ancient intuition quietly shake hands: we are shaped by forces we do not always see, and wisdom is learning how to work with them rather than denying they exist.

Energy: The Ring of Vitality, Metabolism, and Transformation

Energy is not a mood. It is a truth.

In physics, energy is the capacity to do work. In physiology, energy is the currency of every repair, every adaptation, every act of learning. In lived experience, energy is what determines whether insight becomes action, whether hope becomes habit, whether recovery becomes durable.

Biologically, energy lives in mitochondria, glucose metabolism, oxygen utilization, hormonal rhythms, sleep architecture, and the repair cycles that run most deeply when we finally rest. In the brain, energy is expensive. Attention costs. Self-control costs. Emotional regulation costs. This is why people do not "fail" solely from weakness; they often fail from depletion.

In philosophy, energy is will—the animating impulse that makes life more than survival. In depth psychology, it is the direction of desire. In spiritual traditions, it is the lived sense of being alive.

When Energy is out of balance, we see:

- burnout that masquerades as laziness,
- depression that feels like moral failure to the uninformed,
- addiction that becomes an attempt to borrow energy from tomorrow,
- cycles of overdrive and collapse.

To restore Energy is not merely to "motivate." It is to repair the machinery of vitality and then to give it a purpose worthy of its power.

Because energy without direction becomes agitation. Direction without energy becomes frustration. Wellness requires both.

The Rings Are Not Separate: They Interlock

The deeper truth of the Six Rings is that none of them can be "fixed" in isolation.

Air influences Energy; without oxygen and regulation, vitality becomes brittle. Water influences Sound; emotion changes how we hear, how we speak, how we interpret. Earth influences Magnetism; the environments and habits we build determine what pulls us. Sound influences Air; breath follows voice, rhythm follows music. Magnetism influences Energy; alignment reduces waste, misalignment leaks power. Energy influences all of them; depletion distorts everything.

This is why a person can "know better" and still do what harms them. Because knowledge lives mostly in the cortex, while habit lives deeper—in circuits shaped by repetition, emotion, environment, and physiology. The rings remind us that change must be approached as a whole-person phenomenon: biological, psychological, social, and existential.

In the language of systems science, wellness is an emergent property: it arises from the interactions of parts, not from one part alone. In the language of ancient wisdom, wellness is harmony.

Balance Is Not Stillness: It Is a Skilled Return

A final point—perhaps the most important:

Balance is not a permanent state. It is a capacity.

Nature is never perfectly still. The ocean is never "finished." The air is never "complete." The earth itself shifts, seasons turn, storms arrive, droughts pass, new growth comes. To demand unbroken equilibrium from a human being is to demand something even the planet does not offer.

The point of the Six Rings is not to create a life free of strain. The point is to create a life that can *recover*, *adapt*, and *rise*.

In that sense, the Six Rings are a philosophy of resilience:

- **Air** teaches pause and choice.
- **Water** teaches flow and renewal.
- **Earth** teaches stability and nourishment.
- **Sound** teaches resonance and meaning.
- **Magnetism** teaches alignment and protection from invisible pulls.
- **Energy** teaches vitality and transformation.

When these are in dialogue—when none is neglected for

too long—wellness becomes less like a fragile achievement and more like a durable way of living.

And perhaps that is the most hopeful idea of all:

that the forces we search for in healing are not foreign to us. They are already inside us, waiting to be brought into balance—not once, but again and again, as many times as it takes.

THE INSTITUTE OF REGENERATIVE MEDICINE

Published by THE INSTITUTE OF REGENERATIVE MEDICINE • www.irmnfoundation.org/home

This Signature Edition is a compiled and revised volume of the SIX RINGS series. The narratives are composites designed to humanize evidence-based brain wellness and addiction science; names, settings, and identifying details have been altered.

Medical disclaimer: This book is for educational and informational purposes only and is not a substitute for professional medical advice, diagnosis, or treatment. Medication decisions should be made with a licensed prescriber who can consider your history, risks, and goals.

Formatted with Vellum

FDA Disclaimer

This publication is not reviewed or approved by the U.S. Food and Drug Administration (FDA). Any discussion of supplements, protocols, or medications—including possible off-label uses—is provided for educational purposes only and is not intended to diagnose, treat, cure, or prevent any disease. Always consult a qualified clinician for individualized medical advice.

For my boys, Alex and Julian—

You are my steady joy and my quiet strength. Thank you for the laughter that resets the day, the questions that keep me honest, and the love that makes every hard chapter worth writing. Wherever life takes you, may you walk with courage, kindness, and a mind that stays curious.

Chronology Note

This Signature Edition is framed as reflection. John Horacio Harrow's voice is looking back from the COVID-19 era (2020-2021), when uncertainty sharpened old questions about fear, craving, and resilience.

The core events he recounts unfold roughly three decades earlier—between 1994 and 1996—during his early thirties, as he develops the habits of mind that will later define him in *When Dragons Kill*: a physician-scientist's rigor, a forensic scientist's insistence on sequence and evidence, and a human being's unwillingness to abandon hope.

Where the narrative briefly returns to later years (Field Notes), the date is stated explicitly. This is intentional: the book is both a prequel and a blueprint—the developmental foundation for the Privée Clinics ethos and the future John Harrow stories.

Chapter 2

Important Notice

This book is for educational and informational purposes only and is not a substitute for professional medical advice, diagnosis, or treatment.

If you are struggling with alcohol or substance use, or if you are in crisis, please seek help from a qualified clinician, your local emergency services, or a trusted crisis resource in your area.

The stories in this Signature Series are composites and narrative teaching tools intended to humanize evidence-based brain wellness and addiction science. Names, settings, and identifying details have been altered.

Any mention of medications reflects clinical concepts and is not a prescription. Medication decisions should be made with a licensed prescriber who can consider your history, risks, and goals.

Acknowledgments

Foreword

Six Rings has changed the way I view addiction. It is a sickness that can invade the mind. You see how easily those destructive addictions can slip into your life insidiously. Addiction isn't just about "them," the other people. It can affect all of us. Yes, most people consciously know this, however, this book helps you to feel that this is true. It increases your empathy.

In fact, most of us have addictions, some of us are lucky because the consequences of our addictions aren't immediately harmful. But even if you don't consider yourself an addict, you will enjoy this book immensely. Addiction is a result of the brain's workings. We know our brains are important, but we don't take conscious actions or efforts to take care of our precious brain's health. When will we take our brains seriously?

This book looks at all the things self-help books are trying to address by looking directly at the source of it all, the mind.

Prof. Dr. Johnson takes us into the brain, through a journey of fascinating parables, music, art, and science. He shows us how you can improve the health of your brain and use tools to guide your brain to beat addiction, but also to achieve so much more.

Prof. Dr. Johnson has one of the most fascinating brains I have encountered. I have always marveled at his ability to achieve so much with his time. If you see the research that he has done it is impressive and overwhelming. He has utilized and consciously pushed the limits of his own brain in a remarkable way. So I am thrilled that he is sharing some of this knowledge in this book instead of just those close associates, patients, and friends who have had the honor to communicate and learn from him.

Research and academics is one of the many aspects of Prof. Dr. Johnson. His many more dimensions are presented here through his personal stories, creativity, emotional intelligence, worldliness, sophistication, and life adventures. Most people would have to live many lives to experience the same things he has in one life. The combination of his background and experiences and how they interact with important things in our life like, addiction, racism, nutrition, health, science, and religion has created this artistic and musical trip through the brain and addiction. I enjoyed it immensely.

Jessica Johnson Papaspyridis
CEO, Newswise Inc.

Prologue: Train the Mind, Rebuild the Body, Curb Addiction — Before *When Dragons Kill*

When dragons kill, they rarely look like dragons.

In the fluorescent hour before dawn, an emergency department tells the truth without ceremony. A monitor insists on a rhythm. Saline drips with indifferent precision. A chest rises because a machine refuses to give up, and because strangers decide, together, that a life will not be surrendered to a single night.

I have watched addiction arrive in a thousand disguises: polished and employed, exhausted and ashamed, brilliant and terrified. It does not always announce itself with chaos. Sometimes it enters like carbon monoxide, quietly displacing oxygen. Sometimes it enters like a bargain—quietly displacing choice. And sometimes it enters as a personality trait people applaud... until it becomes the only trait left standing.

That is why I use the phrase *When Dragons Kill* as clinical shorthand. Not a fantasy creature, but a learned predator: circuitry strengthened by repetition; craving that becomes fluent; habit that can outpace insight. Dragons kill through ordinary moments: one drink that becomes the tenth, one pill that becomes "one more," one relapse that becomes an obituary.

And yes, the science matters.

Craving is not a moral weakness. It is neurobiology at work: reward, stress, memory, and habit pulling on the same rope. But the human story matters just as much, because neurotransmitters never tell you what it feels like to wake up and realize you have become a stranger to your own promises.

This Signature Edition lives at that intersection—**brain wellness and addiction recovery braided tightly enough that each strengthens the other**. Because addiction is not a "side topic" in these pages. It is one of the book's main engines: alcohol, opioids, stimulants, and the compulsions that mimic them; the myths that keep people stuck; the stigma that makes suffering go underground; and the evidence-based tools that help people return from the edge.

You will meet the **PREPARE Method (Six Rings)**—a framework designed to restore agency without denying biology. It is not a slogan, and it is not a scolding. It is a practical way of seeing:

Preparedness is the courage to name the pattern.

Restoration is the biology of repair.

Evaluative Personalization is the discipline of matching the right intervention to the right person.

Awareness is noticing the first cue, not the last consequence.

Reactivity is choosing a response instead of a reflex.

Elevate is the long arc—meaning, identity, and the life you are rebuilding toward.

But this book also goes where most "wellness" books refuse to go: into the mechanics of *treatment*, including the uncomfortable, necessary truth that for many people, **medications and targeted interventions are not optional luxuries; they are life-saving instruments**. In these pages you will encounter the real-world logic of personalized addiction care: why one person benefits from one approach, and another needs something different; why compliance fails when shame is the hidden co-author; why relapse is often a predictable physiological event rather than a character flaw.

You will see how modern addiction medicine thinks: not “one-size-fits-all,” but **the right treatment, for the right patient, at the right time**—and always, the right dose. You will meet stories that carry the clinical weight of that promise: medication strategies, emerging neuromodulation approaches, and the disciplined humility of clinicians who treat what can be proven, monitor what can be

If you come to this book from *When Dragons Kill*, consider this your origin story: the apprenticeship of attention that eventually becomes an evidence-room habit. And if you begin here, you will meet the man before the legend—before the cases, before the headlines, before the dragons learn your name.

These stories are set decades earlier—**in 1994–1996**—in the years when South Africa was becoming itself again, when history still felt warm from the touch of newly earned freedom. I was in my early thirties then, learning, sometimes painfully, what the body reveals, what the mind hides, and what people will do to avoid feeling what they cannot yet name.

Yet the narrator you hear is older. I look back from the COVID era—not as a claim that these events happened then, but as a time of reflection when the world, newly fragile, forced honesty out of all of us. The events are not rewritten; they are re-seen. That is how a prequel becomes a foundation —not by changing what happened, but by clarifying what it meant.

Medicine asks: *What is happening in this person, and how do we help?*

Forensics asks: *What happened, and how do we know?*

In practice, the questions overlap. A toxicology result is both a clinical clue and a forensic fact. A pattern of injuries can be a diagnosis—and a story of harm. A patient's denial can be a protective reflex, or a missing piece of evidence.

Long before I carried the formal title of forensic scientist, I was already being trained: by addiction, by trauma, by human evasions and human courage, to respect timelines, respect physiology, and respect the difference between what we suspect and what we can prove.

So read this Signature Edition as it is intended: **a health book with the emotional voltage of stories, and the clinical credibility of science**—including the science and treatment of addiction. Read it for the compassion, but also for the precision. Read it because dragons are real.

And because the capacity to train the mind, rebuild the body, curb addiction, and to choose life, again and again, is real, too.

Continuity Interlude: From Clinic to Evidence Room

Chapter 3

Introduction To the Series

Your brain is not a silent organ. It is the living engine of your choices, your hopes, and your future - yet most of us train our bodies more than we train the mind that steers them.

When it comes to alcohol, substances, and the habits that quietly reshape our lives, misinformation is everywhere - while truly effective, evidence-based help can feel hard to find.

Six Rings is a collection of short, story-driven portraits - rooted in real clinical experience, refined through imagination, and designed to bring neuroscience to life.

These stories are meant to be read, felt, and remembered - so understanding doesn't stay on the page, but moves into your day-to-day thinking.

Threaded through each volume is the PREPARE Method (Six Rings): a whole-person approach that honors a simple truth - recovery, wellness, and performance are always personal.

You will also find paintings, music, and imagery used as

mood-setters - small invitations to pause, reflect, and step into the next chapter with fresh eyes.

The author shares his world openly - not to preach, but to humanize the science, to admit complexity, and to remind us that growth is rarely linear.

If these pages spark curiosity, compassion, or courage - if they help you name what you feel and choose what you need - then the book has done its work.

This is not a rigid textbook or a one-size-fits-all prescription. It is a guided journey: evidence-informed, story-rich, and intentionally practical.

Along the way, you will encounter a brief case that foreshadows the anxieties of the COVID-19 era - an example of how uncertainty can grip the mind, and how understanding can loosen its hold.

The PREPARE Method: Six Rings

Chapter 4

Introduction To The Prepare Method

In the winter of 2017, Professor Bankole A. Johnson began shaping a simple question into a workable roadmap: What if we treated brain health the way we treat heart health - proactively, precisely, and with compassion?

The result is the PREPARE Method - powerfully organized, yet designed to be individualized. It is built to meet people where they are, and help them move toward where they want to be.

Also known as the Six Rings, the method interlocks complementary strategies - medical, psychological, behavioral, social, and restorative - so each person has more than willpower to rely on.

To make the ideas easy to follow, this Signature Series presents Six Rings in three books, each one widening the lens and deepening the tools.

Book 1: **P**reparedness and **R**estoration

Book 2: **E**valuative **P**ersonalization

Book 3: **A**wareness, **R**eactivity, and **E**levate

The vision has since evolved into the Privée Clinics model: future global institutes devoted to brain wellness, recovery, and optimization - where science serves humanity.

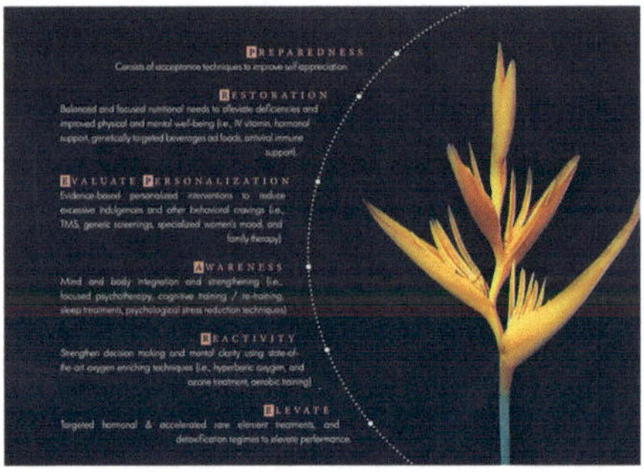

The figure above is: The PREPARE Method (Six Rings) - an overview.

BOOK 1: Preparedness and Restoration

Chapter 5

Introduction To Book 1 of 3

In Book 1, you meet John Horacio Harrow—an ambitious physician-scientist in his early thirties, still learning the costs of brilliance. These stories trace the developmental years that shape the man who will later stand in *When Dragons Kill* as a forensic scientist: precise with evidence, yet fluent in human pain. Even in these early years, he is drawn to the questions that live at the border of medicine and law—the kind that will later place him in forensic laboratories and medicolegal rooms, where compassion must coexist with proof.

John's background is offered as a sketch, not a diagnosis—a lens for how early experiences can shape perception, resilience, and risk.

Born in Africa and shaped by multiple cultures, John carries both pride and fracture from his origins, a reminder that identity is layered, not singular.

School was not a refuge; it was a proving ground. His gifts

set him apart, and the emotional weather at home followed him into every classroom.

He wrestles with expectation, belonging, and a persistent inner pressure. Becoming a physician-scientist was not simply a career choice—it was a way to turn pain into purpose.

By the time many are just beginning adulthood, John is already chasing harder questions: not trophies, but answers—especially for those society overlooks.

His sensitivity becomes his instrument. He notices what others miss: the quiet cues of distress, the hidden patterns of relapse, the moment a person is ready to change.

As brilliant as he is, John keeps learning. He pushes the boundaries of what "normal" health can be—asking not only how to survive, but how to thrive.

This Signature Edition was revised during and after the COVID era, but the backbone of these stories unfolds nearly three decades earlier—chiefly in the mid-to-late 1990s—when John is forging the philosophies that will later become the foundation of Privée Clinics.

In Part One, John confronts his patients' addictions - and his own shadow. You will see how quickly coping can become compulsion, and how compassion can become a catalyst.

In Part Two, the focus turns toward brain wellness: nutrition, restoration, and the everyday foundations that make recovery possible.

The nutritional strategies are presented not as magic, but as support - practical ways to give the brain what it needs to heal, learn, and regulate.

Book 1 also sets the stage for what comes next:

personalization. Because no two brains, no two histories, and no two recoveries are identical.

Take a deep breath. Turn the page. The journey begins.

"...beyond science...beyond borders ***TM****"*

Acceptance

Intellectual Acceptance

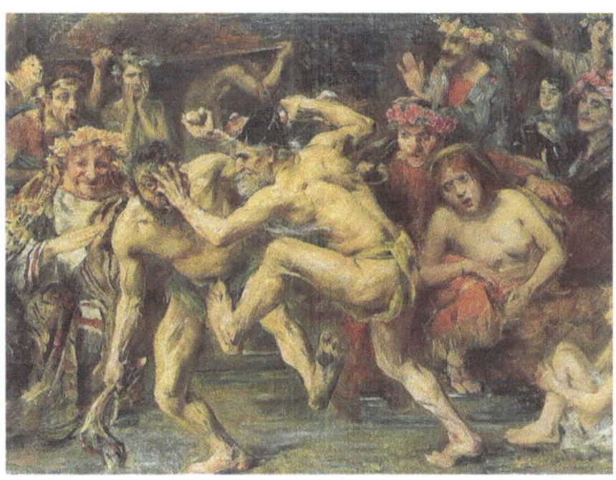

The image above is: Ulysses Fighting the Beggar (1903). Credited to: Lovis Corinth (1858-1925).

In the picture, Odysseus returns to Ithaca disguised as a beggar. The beggar, Arnaeus, stupidly picks a fight with Odysseus and ends up on the floor, grasping for life. [Further credit to]. The allegory to the story is the beggar's fear of being beaten by John.

Sometimes, things are exactly as they seem, but not as they should be.

The early morning sun that glistened on the hood of John's car was reflected by snowflakes into a seeming kaleidoscope of crystals. It was as if miniature cracks were appearing on his windscreen, bursting like raindrops and smearing the view in front of him. Messy, fussy, light indeed. From inside the car, these tiny bursts of light were like rainbows, each dancing to their own tune, never uniting, but producing an aura of foreboding. But this was all light, no darkness - just different hues, playing their tricks to create a mood quite different from how John was feeling that morning.

He looked down at his left-handed, mechanical wristwatch: 7 am. Speeding up would be essential to catching the first meeting early; so, he did. John did not like to be late. For him, 10 minutes late was all that was tolerable. It was the cut-off between running a little late and being careless. John's motto was to be no more than 6 minutes late; 6 being a magical number that exuded calculation rather than tardiness. Six symbolized the power of the hexagon, the strongest natural structure, which had flowed through the sands of time. Any later than that and John felt like the day had been lost. As for being early, in John's mind, that was nothing but plain aggression. It was imposing on another person or being imposed on. Thrusting oneself into another's personal space and time; time being the only elemental occurrence that could not be reversed. Anyone burning time was simply hastening death, and that, by any measure, was not a productive thing to do - dying that is.

At thirty-three, John felt time begin to tighten around the

edges of his days—not as an ending, but as a meter. Every month mattered. Every decision left a residue. In the quiet spaces between appointments, he reminded himself of the simplest truth he knew: there was no higher purpose than the love of family and of God.

John was in a mood that called for "more." He knew that events would shape his day as they gradually unraveled. A day with limited control. He disliked days like this - too imprecise. Yet, resolving to meet each day like a blank sheet of paper, John would wait for the first impressions to yield their true nature. He reached down to the dashboard and increased the volume to full blast. John did not understand why anyone would listen to opera or classical music in the background. It defeated the entire point and was, most likely, a little anti-intellectual. Opera halls went to great lengths to seal all the doors in the days before amplification to create the 'right' sound and mood, just so the audience could feel the music. Why neuter that? What played now was one of his favorite pieces: Maria Callas performing Gaetano Donizetti's Lucia di Lammermoor, come scritto (i.e., as scripted, in F major). So haunting, so moving, so poignant, and so reminiscent of Scotland, with its long history of inter-familial strife, where he had gone to school. And as life meets art, Gaetano Donizetti's own personal life was tragic. He had had three children, all of whom died, and only a year after his parent's passing, his wife followed. All this was too much, and he took ill with a serious mental illness. In 1848, Donizetti died.

Suddenly, it dawned on John why he was in a rotten - perhaps better termed a "rubbish" - mood. He had to attend the funeral of a dear friend later that day. He dreaded funerals. All those people with mixed emotions, and no one having the right words. All attendees, much like at weddings, seemed to him as people in some sort of role-play; with all the customary gestures and conversations being almost as if... scripted. John did not like emotional dishonesty. It pushed the bounds of acceptance into an incredulous world of fantasy. It was a corruption of the soul, and he had been reminded of this in an earlier encounter that year when he had received news of the death of a famous scientist by email and had sent well wishes with a beautiful card to his widow.

Some days later, he got a call.

"Is that Doctor John?"

"Of course. Yes, it is." John had replied.

The widow continued, "I am Martha, Josh's widow. You obviously did not know my husband. He was a horrible man, and a mean drunk, to boot! I waited for decades, hoping he would hit rock bottom and seek help. It never happened. He was the master of near-death experiences, only to be resurrected in a much worse condition each time. I'm glad he's on his way to hades. What a horrible man! Every chance he got, he humiliated me, stole work from his postdocs, their innocence, and..."

John interjected before the widow could continue with the colorful metaphors she was obviously prepared to utter. "I am so sorry, I never knew."

Bang! She had dropped the phone. At first, John was upset. How could she? How could an act of kindness have gone so wrong? But then, he came to have peace with this encounter. Her phone call to him had perhaps done her some good. More so than the card and the nice words, more so than any flowers she may have received, because, above all, she had been intellectually and emotionally honest, which he appreciated. Good for her! This is the path to acceptance. First, we must get rid of all the mush in our heads that is clogging up our emotions, and simply let it all out. The more projectile-like thoughts were, the faster the resolution and cure. Acceptance is a path, a journey if you will, and is not the same for everyone.

John knew he had to get rid of his rubbish mood - for his own sake. Leaving behind these reflections as his car pulled up to a stop sign, he noticed a gaunt-looking man with a lopsided beard approaching him. The expression on his face seemed to deepen the scar he had on his left cheek, and then there was the hobbling gait. It was not reminiscent of any neurological condition that John was aware of. This man was a beggar but perhaps not a real one; simply an opportunist. He was carrying a placard that read:

'*Hungry, need food. Have not had a meal in days. Please help*'.

Turning down the music, John lowered his window. He could not help but to spot the half-empty bottle of spirit in the beggar's pocket and the used crack pipe. Perhaps a good deed would cheer him up, and hopefully, the beggar as well. So, John started a conversation with the beggar.

"I'm John, who might you be, sir?"

The beggar seemed startled and withdrew his outstretched hand. "Uh, my name is John."

Just then, John remembered that his secretary had sent him a text message a few moments earlier to say his 7.30 am meeting was canceled, and he was now not due in until 9.15

am. What a relief. He had been running 11 minutes late - truly a horrifying prospect! Now liberated, John continued.

"Well, hop in, John. I'll take you for breakfast, anywhere you like within a mile."

John had John pre-judged. Handing out dollops of cash to John was not an option. The money would clearly be used to buy more alcohol and drugs. John was having none of that.

"No," John responded. "Capital N-O. I know your type. You just want to kidnap me. Then, thinking no one is looking for me, beat me and discard me like trash. Just give me some money and be gone!"

John knew he had to keep a calm demeanor. This could get serious or even dangerous. This man was definitely not right in the head. John's first thought was, why in the world anyone would think someone who had stopped in broad daylight, at a traffic stop with multiple cameras, would proceed to kidnap a drug-taking, alcoholic beggar on the street? After all, he had been friendly enough. John took a dollar from his center console, handed it to John, and drove off. Now, John was feeling guilty, and still in a rubbish mood. He could not accept that John was a person with free-will but instead concluded his condition had made him a slave of misfortune.

He arrived at the synagogue on time for the funeral. John admired the simplicity of Jewish funerals, and this one was for a dear friend. He had not known him long. But the man had been so loving and warm to John; they could have been brothers. At the service, John heard the Jewish legend of the two brothers who wanted to give selflessly to the other, each believing his brother's crop had been lost.

It was a story of true love! Moreover, it was a tale of acceptance - in all its forms. Acceptance of self, of another person, and above all, acceptance of God. Could life really be that simple?

John reflected. How could his gesture to John, the beggar, have been so badly misinterpreted? John had now discounted any notion that there was something "wrong" with John, apart from being a substance abuser, that is. Allotting the blame to this would've been all too convenient, really. John, being something of a scholar of antiquity, allowed his mind to wander just a bit. He recalled that the idea of a beggar being offered food and then beaten had Hellenic roots. Indeed, in Greek mythology, the role of the beggar was somewhat odd. Beggars who were brought home were invited to beg for food and wine from table to table, with much encouragement. It was as if the beggar was attending a feast all for himself, whereby he would gorge on food and drink. Eventually, some of the hosts would tire of the beggar, and he would be beaten by them. Ergo, the role of the beggar in that instance would be to take the abuse, as some form of catharsis for some of his hosts. At the same time, the role of the beggar was to give thanks to those who had fed him, and to heap opprobrium on those who had humiliated him.

Perhaps, thought John, there was a universal mysticism, or some kind of a *mandala*, or symbolism, that permeated the role of the beggar through cultures, from ancient times to the present, still ending up in a feeding, drinking, and beating cycle.

The mythological role of the beggar could be perceived as one of disguise. Indeed, Ulysses/Odysseus disguised himself as a beggar, so his wife's pursuers would not set upon and kill him. So, even the Gods were aware of the potency and ritual of the beggars' disguise. This chimeric role of the beggar was not to be taken lightly. John knew from his time at Oxford that even the person doing the most mundane of tasks could be a scholar of no modest repute. As a matter of fact, one of the folks who helped collect the rubbish from his tiny apartment at Oxford had been an astrophysicist who had become disillusioned with it all and had sought what he considered a more fulfilling life - working with his hands. John found all this rather fascinating and amusing, albeit puzzling. He sighed. It was like wondering why dolphins became so smart that they just decided to spend all day playing. It was as if there were deeper and spiraling tunnels of understanding in the human mind. That understanding was and is, however, jarred by the expected symbol of "evil." In this case, the protruding bottle of spirit and the used crack pipe wielded by John, the beggar. That defined John's current state, not his intellect, nor anything else that had happened in the past. John felt ashamed of himself. An integral part of self-awareness is reflection, and the best reflections were those where one sees both sides of oneself - like a Janus effect.

Nevertheless, whatever the reason for John's anger at John was, John had worked out that the entire misunderstanding was his, and his alone. And, such an error, to cause someone else to vent such spleen, was probably psychological in nature, and less to do with fables of antiquity.

Then, in an instant, it hit him! It really was quite simple. His offer to help John by the suggestion of food was not perceived by him as a demonstration of love but one of selfishness. The mere act of "feeding" was, in itself, controlling and robbed the recipient of freewill. Control is the opposite side of acceptance and must be resisted if there is to be true self-awareness. Contrasting food, money allowed the recipient freewill to do with it as he or she deemed fit. Here again, the *mandala* was symbolic, money being the gateway to building a platform of acceptance. John also found himself guilty of presumptive arrogance - that John, as if without self-will, would understand his motivation and act accordingly. And also, that he would be fearless, and disregard his own personal safety and get into a car with a stranger. More so, living on the street, John considered, must be the harshest of realities, so nothing could be taken for granted. The amount of disappointment he felt for himself increased.

John knew little about the world of addicts. He had prided himself on not knowing one in his family. How absurd! He was simply either blind or deciding to be blind. Little did John know that the addict also has to reach a point of intellectual acceptance before developing any motivation to seek help.

The next day, at about the same time, John parked his car a block away from the traffic stop. He got out of his car and walked towards John.

"Good morning, John," he began, "I'm so sorry for yesterday. Must have been such a fright for you. Please forgive my arrogance."

John's face lit up, and he placed his hand on John's shoulder. "I'm sorry, too," he replied. "I could have been more polite. I could have given you the benefit of the doubt and accepted your kindness. After all, we are all sons of Zeus.

Please pardon my manners. Six long years out here will do that to you."

Had John just heard 'Zeus,' or was he just imagining it? He looked into John's eyes, the man now seemingly a decade younger, and smiled. Obviously, he had met a kindred spirit in the study of ancient Hellenic traditions.

"Fancy breakfast and a chat then, John?"

"I wouldn't have it any other way."

Now, this would be a better day for both men! Each accepting the other just as they were.

Clinical Note: Acceptance as the First Intervention

A pivotal concept in the world of addiction is acceptance. It is, however, not exclusive to that world but a moniker that the progress from habit to addict skips the point of acceptance that there has been a change. The process seems to also work in reverse. It is the beginning of understanding in the *Rogerian* way of genuineness, giving unconditional positive regard, and accurate empathy [read more]

What fascinates about this concept is that you do not need to be a therapist seeing a patient to utilize it - but it is the same core concept of self-improvement. This philosophy of self-growth transcends formal psychology into the world of meditation and enlightenment. Getting there is different for everyone, but the journey is well worth the trip.

Emotional Acceptance

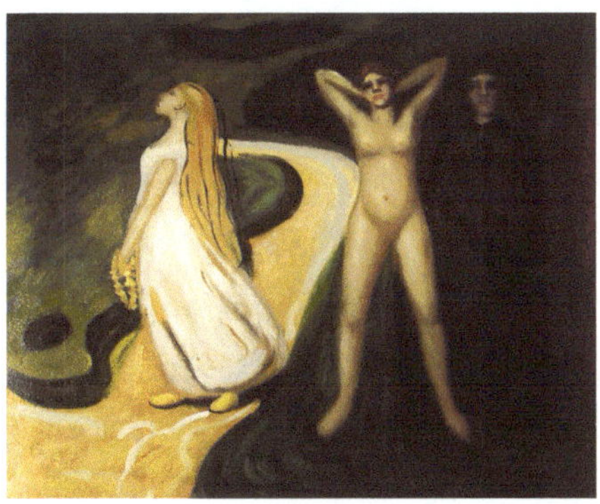

The image above is: Woman in Three Stages (1895) - Edvard Munch.

Emotional acceptance is a deeper connection within an individual that promotes change. This change is in various forms, usually denoted by a path of three steps.

The significance of this artwork to our story is that it symbolizes the progression of various stages of alcohol abuse. The initial state might be said to represent an innocence before excessive drinking ensues. This might be followed by the "fun" stage; a place where the problem has completely manifested but is still assumed to be controllable by the individual and the positive effects are evident. The shadow represents herself shrouded in loss and shame. For the women at the clinic, it involved a process of coming to terms with their entire beings, including the parts which society had taught them to find shameful, so as to eventually triumph over their issues with alcohol use disorder. This is especially important since the cycle of abuse itself was initiated by emotional turmoil. John and Harry also dealt with such a settlement and the need to acknowledge this transformation not just as a phase but a constant journey of self-acceptance and betterment.

In Africa, there is a smell that awakens the senses in the morning.

A warm, musty smell, typical of the bowl of the earth. There was no mistaking it; that is the scent that awoke John. How had he found himself here? He had sworn never again to visit the continent of so much of his sorrow decades ago, yet, he was back!

John climbed out of bed and walked barefoot to the shower. This Africa did not look like the depictions of Africa; this could be anywhere - Miami, London, you name it - except for that distinguishing smell.

John had talked himself into this, or rather, had been talked into it. His mission was simple: to help the locals "cure" or rid themselves of the alcoholics in their town.

In this part of Africa, an alcoholic was a miserable human. A rotten soul with no hope. Nothing could change that. Except here, the so-called alcoholics were mostly women, not men. Many bore children with Pygmalion features; a classic malformation caused by their brew-infused birth type. This was no mistake. It was all, perhaps, because the worst crime towards humanity - apartheid - had deprived the women of their menfolk who were shipped into towns to work. Adding to their pain, they brewed alcohol during the days, waiting for their men to return, and the tasting to perfect the beverage led to more and more drinking, until there was nothing else to look forward to but more and more drinking.

John showered quickly and then powered himself downstairs into a small bus. Eight souls in a small bus... trapped for hours. This was not going to be fun! The man on John's right looked plenty distinguished with a resplendent looking mustache, but his unpolished shoes gave him away. He was no dandy. His grooming was of an urgent tidiness to get over the initial glance, not to impress the deep onlooker. And John was a deep onlooker.

"I am John, and who might you be, sir?"

"Oh, I'm Harry," the man replied, "always have been."

Harry grinned as if to hide some of the pain in his soul. John toyed with asking him more but pulled back. But Harry, sensing a new toy, leaned in.

"Have you ever been arrested, John?"

This instantly disarmed John - did he look like a criminal? But, before he could respond, Harry continued.

"I have. Perhaps about 20 times, maybe more. But do not be frightened. The police enjoyed every minute of it."

Awaiting a follow-up, John anxiously gripped the side handlebars of the bus as it sped along the dusty road. Any question was fraught with danger...and possibly, even more frightful revelations. But he just *had* to ask.

"Why were you arrested so many times?"

"Long story," Harry replied and then winked. It was obvious he wanted to tell this story.

"I was in the freedom movement back in the day, protesting for a color-blind world. Just like now, with you, fighting to help the forgotten and the neglected in this small part of the world."

John nodded politely. He finally realized that he was in a bus full of those devoted to an apostolic cause, not simply "drafted" by an enticing letter, like him. His emotions swelled. How on earth was having a disease like alcoholism a battle that you needed to be freed from? Just didn't make any sense.

Hours swept by as the small bus left the cities behind; the hot afternoon sun beginning to bake everyone. A few of the passengers started to sing, or, more accurately, chant. But this was not any rock song John had ever heard. How he longed to be sitting in his office at home listening to something like Grieg's piano concerto in A minor by Edvard Grieg. Emotionally, this was just the right tune. It was the only concerto Grieg had really completed, and perhaps here, thousands of miles away from the birth of that haunting tune, was the beginning of completion for John. An emotional acceptance, if you like. Like Grieg's concerto, which starts and finishes with a cadenza, so the emotional acceptance in life is like going back to the beginning; and the beginning being like the end. It was a ring of circulating emotion, traveling forward in time, only to return to the same point.

The others in the bus were even less engaging, but

delightful folk beaming with smiles as if on a different mission of exploration. No point engaging them, that might be too scary. John was feeling uncomfortable being in a confined space, surrounded by strangers who all looked familiar, and were all on a conscripted journey. Perhaps this was like being arrested and going to jail.

Was Henry trying to warn me? John mused.

Finally, the bus came to rest, and everyone alighted. It had been a long drive and was much later in the day. John's mind was ablaze with worry.

Would we be stuck here all day...or worse all night?

He couldn't imagine it with these foreign people.

Just as he was beginning to despair, John was greeted by a woman with such a beaming smile. It could only melt away his fear. She was at home and was welcoming him in.

"I'm John," he blurted.

"I know," said the woman he came to know as Harriett, "we have been expecting you. Let me take you to our small clinic."

John walked quickly behind her, leaving most of the others some way in the distance. At least this was some kind of an escape for him.

On entering the clinic, she reached out and said, "here are all my ladies in waiting," just before naming them individually. Her memory was near perfect as she recounted their early lives, their journey, and of course, their pain.

How stupid could John have been? It finally dawned on him. These were not her 'helpers'; these were her clients. But this was no commune, even though their children were everywhere. This was a day clinic, and the women supported each other with childcare.

Much smarter than having someone else you do not know look after your child, thought John.

John knew this was a time to listen quietly, and so did everyone else. The women talked about loss, but mostly of hope. Most of them had been coming to the clinic for several years. John was again surprised. This was not in any textbook he had read or written. The model of alcohol use disorder was of a chronic condition, but these women had turned their disease into a way of life, and in many ways, a journey out of their misery.

Harriett turned to John. He knew this was going to be a question he could not escape answering.

"How do you treat people with alcohol use disorder in the United States? Do they form in groups just like ours? Do they live together?"

This was no easy question, and the truthful answer was itself a revelation. John turned to look at Harry, but he just looked away. Smart man!

So, John started, "Well, it's like this. Yes, we give medicines, and sometimes people go to stay with others for some time, and then, they all get to go home. As for me, I find it unusual to have people live with one another just because they have a disease."

John could not catch the words before they left his mouth, and by the time realization hit, he wished to disappear into any hole in the ground. What he had just said did not even make much sense in this world. All the people he helped were strangers, and even if they came together for a brief time, they departed again as strangers. There was no emotional connection with others in the real sense, and the disease was simply an entity to be dealt with. For the women in this part of the world, alcohol abuse was an emotional symbol, yes of despair and degradation, but also of hope and pride. They had accepted their illness at a deep emotional level and transformed that into their shield. There was a connection between these women and their healing, which was both beyond science and beyond borders. Indeed, it was the power to heal.

Suddenly, it struck John like a bolt. It was one thing to accept at an intellectual level that one had a problem with alcohol; it was quite another to do so at an emotional level. Without emotional acceptance, there was no corner to turn, no value of being, and no real perspective. Alcohol use disorder is not a disease solely related to the amount of drinking, but also to a turning point intertwined between genes and experience, that led to the transformation of the entire individual. Individuals with alcohol use disorder have a myriad of problems other than drinking, and all of this had to be dealt with to bring about a proper path of treatment that endured. Emotional acceptance would allow a transformational change that could now be boosted by medicine. But, medicine alone without acceptance now seemed like a short-term fix. John was humbled. Was it possible that all his training in modern medicine had blinded him to see this first stage of healing? It had always been there in his clients, but he had simply not asked the right questions. The women in this part of the world knew some important truths. Their "change" was not only linked with emotional acceptance, but at its core, a needed reorientation of lifestyle, diet, and social interaction. Here again, the rings that bound the disease within an individual were the same that needed unraveling in a path towards health.

In all of this, John realized that Harry had been quiet, and so had the others. But now, their faces stared at him in concern. Some of them had read John's life story in magazines about never wanting to come back to Africa but were too polite to ask about it.

Harry decided not to try breaking down John's defenses now that he was exactly where he had feared in these nightmares to return. John smiled, everyone smiled, and all left with hugs and a few tears; perhaps, even of joy. No words were said. All that counted was accepting the emotions of the moment.

This emotional acceptance in the group had several steps and differed from one individual to the other. Initially, it had to be recognized, and then some sort of form needed to be put on it. For John, it took traveling into the past, anchored by the music he loved, to recognize and characterize the form. Then, it had to be accepted internally, and finally, there had to be a reflection that brought it all into perspective. For the women he had met in Africa, it had to do with recognizing their problem of alcohol abuse and the many roots of it, organizing it into elements parceled amongst each other, and a period of working together in quiet reflection. The process was the same for both John and the women in its evolution, even though the manifestation differed by the setting and environment. Strangely enough, it also was the same for Harry, who had worked through his pain to reach out and heal. And the other passengers on the bus? Theirs was the power of observation and reflection (what we could name 'empathy') and true positive regard for everyone.

What had he really learned? He had learned to put aside his knowledge and seek to find the "heart" of every client with whom he came into contact. John realized that each of their journeys needed acceptance, not only with the head, but with the heart too, and that bond was the beginning of healing. And yes, there were all those very smart medicines, some of which he had discovered that would help, but there and then, emotionally accepting the client was the beginning...and perhaps ultimately...the circle of the journey towards recovery.

Two weeks later, John returned to the United States.

In March 1996—less than two years after Nelson Mandela took office—John found himself in South Africa as part of a small medical-scientific expedition attached to a U.S. presidential delegation led by President Bill Clinton. Before his return flight that humid afternoon, he ate lunch at a local canteen, trying to let the noise of the room settle his mind before the long journey home.

For the duration of his stay in South Africa, there was ample time for conversation—with Harry, with Roger (a young pharmacist the pair had befriended), and with strangers whose stories carried more truth than any briefing paper.

He wasn't proud to admit it, but left to his own devices, John would rather wait to get back to his hotel to order from the hotel's rather bland all-day English breakfast buffet. It wasn't that good...just familiar, and he needed something of that sort in this strange land.

"You cannot have come all this way and never tried this," Harry would announce, winking. It's an amazing dish called boerewors made of pork and sausage - all wonderfully spiced and infused with garlic. Fatty too - just like your English sausages so you should love them.

"When you are in Rome," Roger would chirp in support.

Between the two of them, John found himself biting into various "Roman" dishes on any of these occasions. On this particular day, though, the associates had somehow turned their attention to the small flat screen towards the front as someone seemed to have increased the volume.

It was nothing positive!

Harry was incandescent with rage - "Racism is truly one of the filthiest conditions a human can have. Sad that those whose minds are poisoned in that way aren't looked at as having some corruption of the soul. Racism should be declared a public health emergency! Then it would get the attention needed so that people of this planet can address and try to fix it once and for all. It's a most serious failure of emotional intelligence" he said.

John looked over at the ever-passionate Harry and exhaled deeply. He was right! The broadcast covered the trial of yet another American police officer being called out for assault and brutality on an innocent black citizen.

"I doubt I could ever live where my color is something to fear or be afraid about," said Freeman, a young black gentleman from England who was sharing a table with them, as he glanced over at his companions who had undoubtedly seen more of the world.

"It isn't fair to stereotype, but...racism exists in every part of the world, even in England" said John.

John relaxed his focus on the events unfolding before him

and considered both sides of the issues. He had so many good friends, colleagues, clients of different races who would be just as horrified by such actions, but he couldn't pretend hate didn't exist either.

John had a unique vision of racism, which he seldom shared. For him, the way to combat racism was not only in marches or protests but in economic activism. If only people of color did their research and only supported businesses with a history of equality, matters would surely change. Also, he thought that the persistence of organized racism in some Whites was not only a lack of education, but also that they too need to be freed from the original sin of slavery. But who was there to do that? What role model was there who would instill so much respect as to champion peace, love, compassion, and reconciliation? Who could teach emotional intelligence on a national scale except a respected leader, and where was he or she to be found?

John had greeted the news in May 1994—that South Africa had elected its first Black president—with a kind of hope that felt almost physical. It stirred his sense of justice, and it deepened his gratitude for the country that had naturalized him and taught him to keep turning toward evidence, not fear.

The shock of seeing the news reports from America come to life was something he hadn't been prepared for.

In America, from the attitude of suspicion John had initially been regarded by his White patients, to the general doubt of his abilities, mundane parts of life carried underlying tones of prejudice. John recalled his first real taste of racism when one of his tutors, hearing of his scientific successes, and misguidedly wanting to congratulate him, had written to him, describing him as a "genius" only to add that he felt sorry for him as he was really a "White man trying to get out of a black man's skin" How humiliating! Racism is not a jail you get out of simply by status. John, now a roaring success, never really encountered this type of brutal racism anymore, and worried that he had lost touch in the vanilla of just "fitting in" - at least most of the time.

On another day during that same trip to South Africa, he entered the canteen with Harry and Roger, and something on the wall caught his eye—an old message, barely painted over, that still managed to speak.

Whites only

After being ignored by servers in the disorderly line for several minutes, a petite, blond server had sidled straight up to him and simply made eye contact for some seconds.

"Do you know that if it not for all that's going on, a month ago, you couldn't have even set foot in here? And, if you'd managed to, you would've had to use the servants' restroom?"

Giving him another once over, she left just as suddenly, muttering under her breath. A strange feeling of inadequacy washed over him. John recoiled and transfixed his gaze back to the television as his companions attempted to shift the conversation to lighter matters. Images of impassioned protesters wielding their black and white placards flitted past the screen.

John did choose to see the world as a better place, but for now, there was another immediate cause he needed to support once he returned home.

A Lack of Emotional Intelligence and Its Consequences

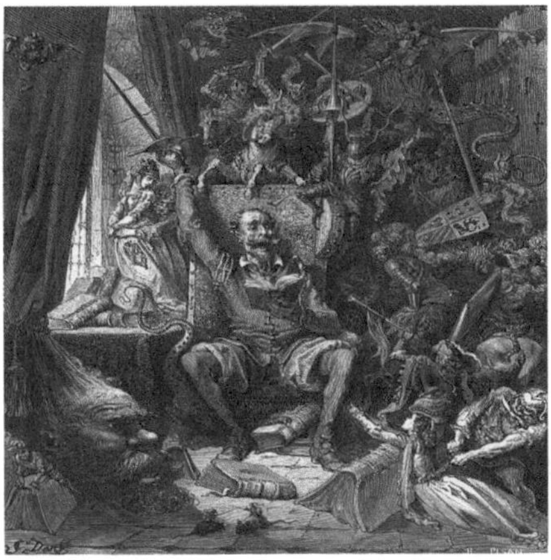

The image above is: Gustave Doré's depiction of Don Quixote (engraving; frontispiece to the 1863 Paris Hachette edition).

Like the celebrated tale of Don Quixote, the protagonists in this story are on a chivalric quest to get back to their loved ones (John to his pregnant wife and Harry to his girlfriend) and will seemingly let nothing stand in their way. Their battles against the elements and themselves is allegorical to Don Quixote's struggles in the novel by Miguel de Cervantes. Are John and Harry enjoined in a relationship akin to Don Quixote and Pancho Sanza? Did our protagonists get away with their deeds or suffer a similar fate? Or worse?

I refuse to die in bed, John muttered to himself.

He was not sure how this thought had entered his head, but it related to a dream he had of how a man who lived next to a railway station had been so fearful of being killed by a train that he never left his house. Somehow, life would throw an unexpected turn, a train had derailed, and he was killed anyway. Bad dreams portend an even worse day.

The morning did not start like any other, although his plans were clear; get out of the office ahead of a snowstorm, catch the last flight out from Richmond to Atlanta, and then, on to London the next day to be in the arms of his wonderful and now, pregnant new wife. What could be simpler? John had made this trip several times before and did not even need to think about the steps.

But the snowstorm had started early. John decided to take a limo to the airport. As the limo fishtailed its way to the Richmond airport, he knew every second counted. 30 MPH on a motorway - and that felt fast too. John arrived 26 minutes before departure...and that set an entire cascade of events and poor decisions into motion.

There are always three of these emotional decision points that matter in a crisis, and John was about to face the first one.

Busy check-in attendants are seldom nice. This is most

likely due to a mixture of too much lousy airport food, and a hostility borne from a job that never appears to have a deadline. John had a visual nightmare of the attendant's cognitive processes. It went something like this: The plane's leaving in 5 minutes, so why on earth should I not take 10 minutes to check-in the next traveler, then send him on a hopeless mission against time? Even though there would be the frustration of the teeming mass that re-appeared to reschedule, she would take pride in being able to tell the "I told you so" lesson on the spot, and better still, revel in quoting regulations that defied common sense in the situation that had emerged; an evil trap that never failed to forestall the most amicable but now frantic traveler. It was the ultimate and most unvarnished example of schadenfreude.

John snapped out of his daydream as the attendant began to work her mischief.

"Sorry, I cannot check your luggage in," the woman said in a middle-class British accent.

John had met her sort before. Her haggard face bore the disappointments she had suffered in love - this being primarily her fault - and now, obviously bitter, she derived her happiness in pouring out her bile on any middle-aged man who might be the type to have jilted her. She looked older than her age, and every ounce of pain her words inflicted made the corners of her mouth curl and made her face deepen. This was the perfect description of ugliness; that which emanated from a barren soul.

"The regulations say I cannot check you in 25 minutes before departure. You can go, but your luggage will have to stay. Homeland security regulations, you know."

"But we are earlier by 25 minutes! There is a snowstorm, and we shall be lucky to get out of here in an hour," John reasoned. "I have to get back to my pregnant wife. It is our first child, and I am so excited." And he looked it.

This, however, only seemed to egg on the attendant, who responded, "Well, that was a minute ago, and let me please repeat myself..." and then proceeded to do so in a sarcastic tone that only certain types of British people can muster. It went along the lines of; state the obvious louder and slower, in the hope that the Americans, who had but borrowed the language, would understand.

John hated this kind of arrogance. He was proud to be both American and British, but how would she know?

Without the Americans, he thought to himself, *we* might all have been spending time in a lovely German concentration camp right now. But there was no use telling her that. John knew that he was defenseless against this type of authoritarianism. His resistance and reasoning would just have elicited no different sentence, adding to his own fury by so doing. Alluding to his education at one of the finest universities on earth would, simply, have evinced her anger, contempt, and disdain, followed by a statement to the tune of "a man of your education really should know better". While mockery would have sent her into an unintelligible diatribe. Time was short.

John backed down, gave the luggage to the limo driver to return to his home, and ran for the gate. This was not going well. He could not have known that this was only a hiccup in comparison to what was coming!

Last call for Atlanta.

"Get a move on, man, we are all waiting for you," the gate attendant said.

"Sorry, I am doing all I can," John said. "Hard to move my bones at my age," he continued.

"I have a coach seat for you, sir," she informed him.

"May I please just have the business class seat I paid for?"

"I will have to check if that is possible," she stated.

"Can a manager help you?" John inquired in a slightly threatening manner.

Sure enough, once the manager came over, the business class ticket was printed, and in a jiffy, John was nestled in his seat. Why is a manager always needed to do the obvious? He could not wait to get home to London.

The plane was caked in ice. The blizzard had started, and the wind had picked up a ghostly howl. John reminisced about a similar encounter on the East Coast in the winter of 1996 on just as much of a snowy Armageddon. Those were the good old days, before 9/11 when the only enemy was the elements and the usual mix of incompetence. On that day, he had managed to annoy the captain of a domestic flight by getting pizza delivered on board, then selling it at $50 a slice to his hungry co-passengers in business class who the crew had refused to feed for 6 hours. He had made an excellent profit on his investment, and so did the pizza delivery boy. How did John do this? He knew, so he thought, one or two things about his fellow humans. They would always answer a gentle knock at the door, especially if they did not know who was on the other side. The flight attendant had opened the door, and in the confusion of trying to decide what to do, John had got the pizza in his hand and had started handing out the pre-sold portions. The defeat of useless bureaucracy is always a thrilling pursuit, not because it requires bravery, but because it pitches guile and cunning against - you guessed it - following more useless rules and regulations. The victory that day belonged to John! But, today was another kind of day.

This day was not going to plan.

John had watched too many airline disaster documentaries, and this felt like the prelude to one of them. All the necessary elements were present: confusion, bad weather, and a pilot determined to do vicious combat with Mother Nature. His plan seemed simple enough: de-ice the plane, get to the runway, and take off. If only practice followed planning precisely. Perhaps in a perfect world, that would be so. But his present world, at this precise time, was far from perfect.

The intercom crackled. "Here is your captain from the flight deck..."

Where else would he be? John's salty thought cut in.

"The runway is so packed with ice that by the time the snowplows reach the end of the runway, there would be so much snow in front that take-off would be impossible. I plan to taxi behind the plows, and as they get to the end of the runway, accelerate and then take off."

This was not a man who read books about regulations! This was Dan Dare, Buck Rogers, and Captain Kirk; all rolled into a single individual. John ordered a Bloody Mary and reflected that if this was it, if this was THE end, what would his greatest regret be? That was fairly obvious: staying in a loveless marriage for 17 years, and worse, marrying someone just like the check-in attendant.

But now, all was well. He had met the woman of his dreams, and they were having a baby - life was great.

Hold that thought! If this were his last memory, then he would thank his Lord!

Now, John was terrified. The first of those three emotional decision-points he had earlier recalled had arrived. What was there to do, though? Scream and insist on being taken off the flight, fake an epileptic seizure, or just accept his fate? He decided to accept his fate. Not like a lamb, but in full consciousness that incompetence could not only seal his fate but could also come to his rescue.

And then, it happened. The snowplows crashed into one another, sending debris everywhere - take-off aborted. Squash the thought that it was John's plane that had careened into the snowplows. The ghoulish excitement was palpable in the cabin. Cell phones were switched on, and 200 or so strangers called their loved ones to revel in their lucky escape.

"Be home in a few hours. I shall slip into bed, and you can kiss me in the morning," went one passenger's call. But it was not over. The pilot, however, was just getting started.

"This is your captain again. I have asked for the debris to be cleared (John was waiting for him to say 'bodies'), but now I am out of fuel (and if that had happened midair?). I shall go back to the terminal, get more fuel, de-ice again, and try to take off on another runway with different snowplows. I am not canceling this flight. I need to get out of here just like you folks."

Tension rose in the cabin. Now, even John agreed that one thing trumped incompetence. It is what the British called "bloody stupidity," with Americans more politely referring to it as a failure of common sense. This was a shining example of it if he ever saw any. This was not going to end well! Now was the time to fake that epileptic seizure. Just as John rose to the occasion, the intercom boomed again.

"Sorry to disappoint you, folks, the control tower have canceled the flight, and I cannot do anything about it. I was willing to try."

John sighed in relief. Thank God there was someone who had read those useless regulations (or the lack of them) just when it was needed! But had the same emotionally unintelligent virus that afflicted our captain unwittingly infected John? We shall see.

What was wrong with just trying to get out the next day? A rush had turned into an urgency that had resulted in an emotionally pregnant emergency, which then gave birth to a crisis of emotions. A Kafka-like spiral of poor emotional decision-making, with no off-turn to do the reasonable thing. The invented crisis, stemming from that first poor emotional decision to rush rather than accept what was the more discerned thought, was deepening. It is the same with an addiction, the first sip of a drink or the first use of the drug comes with a compelling thrill, only to be followed by a series of poor decisions, outcomes, and ultimately, suffering!

Now the race was on to the car rental. Just in case there was a long line of those who also wished to drive through a blizzard. Nothing could really be left to chance.

"You can have this Lexus SUV," the rental agent said.

"But Madam, I want a real American SUV," John quipped.

"It is a real SUV, sir. 4-wheel drive, top of the line, and our premium model," she replied.

"Fine, I will take it," he accepted.

Now, for the nineteenth law of business: take advantage of a desperate customer.

"That will be $350/day plus taxes, and have a nice day," the agent concluded.

That was when John met Harry, and his real journey began.

Harry had been interviewing at a nearby university and simply had to get back to Florida to meet his beloved, who was waiting for him at a swanky hotel he had booked. He fidgeted.

John spoke up to the nervous-looking man.

"How would you like to drive with me to Atlanta? We could skip all the rebooking tonight, and drive in the morning. We can give ourselves 12 hours to drive to Atlanta, stay overnight, and lose just one day. Because everyone is still stuck here, and presumably, most of everywhere else on the East Coast, I guess we could have our choice of bookings from Atlanta?"

Harry looked this stranger over for a minute. After calling to discuss this proposal over the phone with his girlfriend, he agreed. They were on their way. The plan was to stay at a hotel 30 miles south of Richmond to get a little away from the heaviest mix, and then start out at 9 AM. There would be a break in the weather before noon. That was when they would make a run for it! In the best of worlds, all this haste and fury had a slim chance of success, compared to just waiting a day. To them, their actions would save a day, but they were soon about to unravel unforetold dangers and emotional exposures instead.

The next day started well even though they had arrived at

the hotel at about 2 AM. Harry was waiting for John at breakfast by about 8:15 AM. They both ordered eggs and bacon, the warriors' breakfast, and were all packed and ready to go at 9 AM. This plan was on target.

"Better hurry," warned the checkout clerk at the hotel. "It is coming back in, and you will be here for days if it catches you here.

For a survival kit, they grabbed two bottles of water and Kit-Kats and waved goodbye.

The roads were absolutely terrible! 15 MPH was like being in a racecar at full speed, and mostly sideways. Then, John made the decision that changed everything.

"Harry, can I swing by my house in Charlottesville to make sure I have not left the heating on, and then we will blast down to Atlanta?"

"Sure," his companion agreed, and that single word joined both men in their fate for the next 24 hours.

That was the second point of three in the emotional launch into crisis. Why had Harry not simply asked John how he had arrived at that thought? Was it fear or anxiety to challenge a stranger? Sometimes, the anxiety of not asking the obvious, simple question can spell doom.

Bad decisions are easy to spot in hindsight. When they unfold before your eyes, you'd know it really was a terrible decision. Abandoned cars on the side of the road, walking motorists, and no snowplows marked where they were going.

"Where on earth do you live?" Harry asked.

"In the countryside. We will be there soon," John replied.

This was not entirely true. They were still 8 miles away, John's steering wheel was a blur with all the corrections he had to make, and he knew that pressing the brakes, or stopping for the single red light that he would encounter, would doom them to staying at a shelter over the weekend. Somehow, John made it to his front gate and applied the brakes. The car skipped and then stopped. They were stuck! Snow piled up to the height of the car's door, which was facing the wrong exit direction.

"We are truly fuck**d!" Harry exclaimed. "We will never make it. This is so bad!"

"Be positive," John answered in an infuriatingly calm manner as he clambered out of the car.

One of John's ancestors in heaven must have been playing the theme song from the Dam Busters. John loved the tune, but more importantly, it swelled his heart with pride to think that, as a groundbreaking scientist with dozens of global patents to his name, he too was a Dam Buster. The British are, simply, glorious people!

He snapped out of his daydream to find his neighbor, driving his green tractor, apparently racing to their rescue. The men pumped their fists.

"I told you to be positive," said John. Unbeknownst to him, their movie had only just started.

John's neighbor was one of those people who are simply the salt of the earth - rugged, kind, big hands, and spit-chewing tobacco.

"Let us get you out of here," he said. The man may not have looked like a superhero, but he was to them. An American hero extolling all the virtues of forbearance, persistence, to the point of making sacrifices to help his fellow man or woman.

Then, John made a decision that would shape his mindset for the rest of the day; he would get into the house one way or another to switch on the heating. Who has thousands of dollars to spend for the repairs of a frozen, and later, burst pipe? Starting out while his neighbor's back was turned, he soon fell into a ditch. John was waist-deep in snow and sinking fast. Screaming proved useless as no one could hear him; the tractor was too loud. In 30 seconds, he would be under, and in some minutes, completely gone. Surely, this is not how it ends? The embarrassing headlines would read:

World-famous scientist drowns to death in a ditch.

This was a pivotal moment. A wrong turn could be fatal. Now, this was the time for John to use that brain of his to survive. Then, the idea came to use all the remaining energy he had to flip as much as possible on his front to increase his surface area. Yes, he would go down faster if that failed, but, hopefully, his large visage would leave a crater large enough to raise his neighbor's curiosity to investigate in a minute or two. He would try to hold his breath, and if that did not work too well, John would create small air pockets by eating ice. He hated the stuff, but there was no time for a pilot study. Now, John was on his belly, still sinking fast, but paddling like fury with his arms. Luckily, he hit the edge of the ditch with his right hand and managed to haul himself up slowly.

Covered in mud and snow, he was simply glad to have survived.

"Doing OK?" his neighbor asked after shutting down the tractor.

What would have made John's death even more futile was

that the heating in the house was already on. How would his meaningless demise be explained to his ancestors in heaven?

Back in the car, and only a hundred feet down the road, they are stuck again. John's neighbor informed them he would have to go for help, and this would take about 10 - 12 minutes. They thanked him and waved goodbye, not knowing that this would be the last they would see of him that day, but that would be their own fault.

An hour later, Harry was getting restless.

"We cannot sit here all day. We need to try and get out." John agreed.

They took turns rocking the car backward and forwards, and eventually, they were free! But not for long. Another 200 meters along, and now out of sight of the first place they had been beached, they found themselves stuck again. This time, they were stuck right in the middle of the road.

How easy is it to confirm one's prejudices? As one monster truck after another with a confederate flag in the rear window rolled past without even slowing to offer help, Harry simply had to repeat his previous question: "Where on earth do you live?"

This time, an inspired response was needed. "Next to one of the richest estates in the world, and a stone's throw from the home of 2 ex-Presidents. This is Virginia."

Harry was not impressed.

Now, for a better plan.

"Harry, why don't you stand in the middle of the road, and flag someone down as best you can. I shall stay in the car. Offer them $100, with the promise of more, to tow us to the highway?" John suggested.

But, Harry had a moment of insight. "I think you should do this."

"Glad to," John replied.

The first person they got to stop was a tall, lanky man with a ginger beard.

"I have been pulling cars out all day, and I need to get my new puppy home," he replied hastily.

"We can offer you an incentive to get us out of here. I need to get to my pregnant wife, and my friend here needs to get to Florida," said John, trying to bargain with a bribe or through empathy.

This is not working. John decided to up the stakes. "Hell, I'll just buy your truck," he boomed.

While some say money is not the answer to all problems, there is definitely something suspicious about a man who cannot be persuaded by sentiment, pity, or cash. They were dealing with a renegade. His soft voice had masked his true nature. Some time ago, John watched a movie like this where some people had been stuck in the woods. It was called The Deer Hunter, and it did not end well.

"The best help I can offer is to push you off the road so that I can get by," the ginger said.

Harry thought this was a great idea. John knew better. His plan was to push us off the road so he could get by. Plain and simple. There was no help involved. Having worked this out, John muttered to Harry.

"If we are by the side of the road, no one would help. By blocking the road, at least no one can now truly get by without stopping."

But Harry was a gentleman. "That would not really be fair."

John was growing exasperated. "Life and surviving are not fair," he retorted.

"Let us trust him," Harry said. So, they did.

Sure enough, as soon as they had been moved aside, the man drove past in his truck and did not look back. At that moment, John glanced in the rear-view mirror. His neighbor with the tractor was in the distance, but he could not see them because they were now pushed off the side of the road. But he had come back and kept his promise! How ironic! Both the best and worst of human nature were playing out simultaneously right before their eyes.

Plan B!

"Alright, let us call the rental company, tell them the car is now abandoned and get them to come and get us out of here with a tow truck," John said to Harry, "while implementing Plan C simultaneously; call 911, state we are stranded, blocking the road, our health could deteriorate, and we need help," he finished.

Harry thought neither plan was worth doing. The emergency services would be stretched. They would not come. The men could sit there for ages, or worse, freeze to death, waiting for rescue.

John felt like this was the opportune moment to launch his first pep talk. "Harry, everything will be fine. We must stay positive, think of plans, and implement them. No good will come of just sitting here. I am sorry about my bad decision to come here, but now that we are here, let us work to fix it. Think of your girl in Florida, and the first thing you would like to do when you see her."

"Okay. You make the calls," came Harry's hesitant reply.

Both calls were placed. ETA for either rescue was 3 - 4 hours. Back to plan A.

"Harry, let us keep trying to flag someone down to help us," John said.

About an hour later, a kind man named CJ and his wife stopped to help. He wanted no money but promised to come back and tow the stranded men to safety. True to his word, CJ did return. However, in the interim, John had persuaded someone else to stop and pull them back to the center of the road. Now, they were back to blocking the main road. Now, someone had to help! It did not hurt that they could be seen for miles. The problem was, for CJ to tow them forward, he had to get by them, risking falling into a ditch himself with his truck. CJ took the chance, but luck was not on his side. He almost tipped over.

Now they were both stuck! John reflected on the story of the Good Samaritan in the Bible. As a child, he was taught this story as a man helping a robbed and beaten traveler, a foreigner and stranger to him at the time. What John had failed to grasp in that story was the underlying moral lesson. Being a Good Samaritan carries a severe emotional and physical risk, probably even higher than that of the person being helped. It also required selflessness, which is the best we humans have to offer our galaxy. It is a story of the best of us, and ultimately of faith in ourselves. The men tried in vain to help CJ, but his car was damaged, his spirit dimmed, and he was possibly facing an expensive repair. CJ had reached out to some of his own friends to come and help, but they had turned him down. His faith in human nature was diminished. That is when John posed his moral dilemma to Harry and the third of the emotional turning points that can happen in a crisis.

"Harry, the ice is melting a bit, and there is a chance we may get unstuck because we are on the main road. But if that happens, we cannot stop and help CJ. We will have to keep going and leave him stranded. His cell phone could fail, and then he cannot call anyone for help. He would be alone. Do we stop and remain with him or keep moving?" John expounded.

"That will never happen," Harry simply replied.

Well, they were about to be tested!

Somehow, their car came unglued. They were moving, and now John was hard on the gas.

"Stop, we are leaving CJ behind!" screamed Harry.

But, his companion was firm. "We are not stopping! We had the chance to debate this moral dilemma an hour ago, and you dodged the question. Now the moment of choice is upon us, and I have decided for you."

The escape route was dangerous. There were a few light tracks on the road (probably left by the monster trucks), but they were on the wrong side of the road.

"Harry, one more thing, I am driving on the opposite side of the road, I will not swerve. Any car coming to us will have to swerve or run into us headlong. My calculation is that the only cars that we will meet will be huge trucks and they will swerve because they can," was John's announcement.

"You are crazy! We will be killed!" Harry exclaimed.

"You took a ride with a man you did not know, and agreed to drive with him for almost 500 miles in a snow blizzard; which one of us do you think is crazy?" John snapped.

Accurately enough, cars coming towards them moved over.

Unknown to Harry, John was praying to God to help them, and for his ancestors to come to their aid, and for a miracle to happen. And the miracle did happen! At least, for a while.

As they drove past CJ, John had the presence of mind to throw his cell phone at him, which the new captive caught. It was the least they could do. If this were a quiz on emotional intelligence, they would have received a failing grade. They really should have discussed all the possible outcomes with CJ and included him in the decision-making process.

They were back on their way and were heading to the motorway. But, CJ was still stranded, even though he now had John's cellphone to call for help. How fair was that? Harry inquired of John about the fairness of the situation. John told Harry that he should also consider all the military personnel returning home from the war on their two-week break who could not get home - wives and husbands worried, children crying, and friends and loved ones depressed at the destination airport. They had given up seeing their loved ones for the war effort. They had survived, but now, fate had taken a cruel turn and robbed them of re-unification. How fair was that? The truth is that there is no right answer to misery, and no wise words can pour solace on this type of heartbreak. John and Harry were sad for those soldiers, giving so much for everyone, yet relatively unnoticed. They bowed their heads in utter humility to honor the men and women who sacrificed.

It should be noted that the police that was sent to help, who had ended up asking that they walk towards them for 3 miles to be rescued, did not show up. How could the uniformed services of this country be so different? John had quashed Harry's suggestion that they do what the police dispatcher had requested. Not because of mistrust for the police but simply because he had no intention of sleeping in a homeless shelter. In hindsight, he was pleased with himself for having made that decision. They might have died of hypothermia wandering in the woods in the middle of the night with no one there, no food, and no water.

Eventually, they were able to reach CJ by calling John's phone and confirmed he was safe. CJ had used the phone to call his wife, who had fetched him. He wanted no money. Most likely, he did not think much of them. They assured CJ's wife that they also had used Harry's phone to call the emergency services and alerted them that CJ was there, as well as diverting the tow truck from the rental company that had been sent for them towards him. But alas, she had got there first. They offered to pay for all the damage to his truck and wished to invite them to John's home on his return. They hoped he understood their predicament and asked for him to forgive their selfish decision. CJ's wife was really nice to Harry on the phone and reassured him that all was well. However, Harry was left with a heavy heart as to whether his decision had changed CJ forever. This is the problem with moral dilemmas; the urgent reality is nothing like having to live it out in regular life. They pressed on!

Their tribulations were not yet over.

The motorway was strewn with stranded vehicles. Some with their lights still on, so they knew the occupants were still inside, hoping to be rescued. Harry turned and looked at John, who had seen that look of despair before.

"We will never make it. Not ever, not in this sh**ty Lexus. It's fairly clear now that it isn't really a 4-wheel drive, just a 2-

wheel," Harry complained. It was not the car's fault they picked up the wrong specification of the vehicle. He was almost in tears.

Now was the time for the second and third pep talks all rolled into one. "Harry, the situation is desperate, and our chances are not good. But that does not change a thing. That is why we are here - to meet our challenges. We shall succeed. Be positive. I never give up. Not now, not ever. I never second-guess myself," he said, as they hurtled towards Roanoke...and yet another crisis.

Roanoke was backed up close to 100 miles. Harry had called his girlfriend, who had confirmed parts of the motorway were blocked. They were not going anywhere. And they did not for almost 2 hours. John asked Harry to call their hotel in Atlanta to cancel. Their only hope would be to drive through the night if this ever cleared. Restroom facilities beside the motorway had no privacy, but they had to make do. It was interesting to observe how quickly the veneer of our civilization could start to peel back in just a few hours of the external pressure of adverse climatic conditions.

When they started to move, it was treacherous. 20 MPH felt like high velocity, and at every turn, there was the danger of falling off the road. Many did. They were in their very own disaster movie. Who would pay to watch a movie entitled Escape from Roanoke?

The further they crawled along, the lower Harry's spirits became. He was desperate. Eventually, even suggesting they stop over at a Days Inn, despite it being in the middle of nowhere because it had a heated indoor pool where he could clean off and get warm. They would sleep and wait out the storm. John reminded Harry that the former had met the woman of his dreams. She was pregnant with their baby, and he was not going to miss the first ultrasound in 2 days. If Harry wished to go to the Days Inn, that would be his decision, and John would have to leave him there with his luggage.

John spent a couple of hours explaining to Harry that his own life had been a journey of perseverance, and of struggle. Ultimately, he made his own decisions. Granted, John was not always right, but some of the choices were his also. He told Harry that for him, decisions of commission, even if wrong, were better than ones of omission and regret.

For his part, Harry was an upper-middle-class man of Jewish background. He had had a traditional Jewish upbringing and could hear his grandparents screaming "stop" every time he got too close to the edge. Now, he was chained to a maverick in a deadly winter storm. Harry was a reliable friend and a wonderful family man, never getting into any real trouble in life, but rather, leading it quietly and with as much dignity as possible. He was the type of man who would drive 8 MPH over the speed limit, but ask him to do 10 MPH over, and he would snap into a panic. He was the type of man most fathers would wish their daughters to marry. But John was not marrying Harry to his daughter; he was simply his companion on an arduous and dangerous journey. The requirements were rather different.

After John's unpaid psychoanalytic session, Harry asked what had shaped the more resilient man's personality and what the perfect personality was. The former assured Harry that his own personality was also far from perfect. Indeed, it was incomplete and mostly flawed. John confided in Harry that if he had a twin brother, they would probably not get along well. His personality suited change, invention, and resourcefulness. John struggled against boredom and impatience, marveling at the wisdom of some of his own tutors. The price he sometimes had to pay for his personality was loneliness. He did not have many friends, but the ones he did have were like treasures to him. John would do all he could for them. He always listened to his inner child, and that enabled him to advance with confidence. Having descended from a long line of warriors and pioneers, one of his ancestors was fabled to have been so fierce and determined that when he was beheaded in battle, he reached out for one of the other heads on the ground, placed it upon his neck and continued fighting. The warrior's wife never slept with him again when he returned home, as she regarded him as an ugly imposter. This is part of the folklore of John's native country told to many young children. One day, he hoped to be worthy of that legacy.

John told Harry to quit all his talk of dying. When that time came, his ancestors would be there to help him. They were still pressed on. He told Harry that he would be prepared to be a mentor for him should he wish it.

They got past Roanoke, and now, the battle was against time and high winds. Heavy gusts blew across Charlotte, and the only respite came when they hit South Carolina. From there, it was a countdown. Harry tried to reschedule his 7:35 AM departure, but the travel agent duped him. Telling him to call back 30 minutes later to be assigned a seat following his initial call, but in the interval, giving his seat to someone else.

Harry seemingly did not insist strongly enough. John had done all he could to help his new friend. 90 MPH in high winds in a small SUV is not what anyone would call fun. There were many 'wow' moments.

Finally, they arrived at Atlanta airport, about 45 minutes before Harry's scheduled departure. He alighted, and John told him to run to the terminal to get into his lover's arms. He would return the car to the rental company. It had been a 24-hour road trip. John got back to the terminal after completing his task and began to check in. He joined the queue in front of a new recruit who had just finished basic training. John asked him his name and thanked him for his service.

The recruit simply replied, "Alexander."

John looked on gratefully. "If my first child is a boy, I shall call him 'Alexander'."

Unfortunately, his heavy computer case slipped and fell on the recruit's foot. John apologized amply.

"Do not worry. I cannot feel my feet anymore. It has been so cold, the nerves in them must be dead."

John thanked him again for his sacrifice, booked his flight, and eventually arrived safely in London the next day. As the plane took off, John had screamed to himself on the inside:

I refuse to die in bed!

Epilogue: an explanation of the tale

This is an allegorical tale to highlight how a series of poor emotional decisions and non-acceptance can be associated with addictive behaviors.

Key to this tale: there are many turning points presented in which the protagonists could have chosen to withdraw from their situation, but instead, pressed on down a spiral. All the jump-off points were ignored or argued at from an intellectual instead of an emotional standpoint. This tale also highlights how prejudices can deepen a mindset such that it becomes impossible to "hear" any alternatives. The case of the Good Samaritan is used to emphasize that sometimes even helpers can be put at risk. Throughout the tale, there is a feeling of desperation and decline, which the protagonists are mostly responsible for, but cannot see a way out of themselves. This has parallels with addictive behaviors in which the individual is often intellectually aware that a better decision can be made. Still, the emotional burden of the disease prevents this different option from being taken. Even though the tale ends with success and their aim being achieved, John remains defiant. This reflects the true nature of addictive behaviors, in that the brain's best decisions are hijacked in the pursuit of a singular and overwhelming goal, which in this case, was the protagonists reaching their destination. The relationship between John and Harry is intriguing. Even though Harry is a 'good man', his unwillingness to challenge John's wild ideas makes him an accomplice. In the realm of addiction, Harry would come across as an "enabler" who seemingly wishes to please; his inability to ask even the most obvious questions making him complicit in the outcome.

There are critical elements that define low emotional intelligence. Some of those depicted in this tale include John's aggression, selfishness, stubbornness, and being critical of others. Harry displayed some aspects of high emotional intelligence like predictability and stability but lacked others that would have been helpful, such as; assertiveness, persuasiveness, and being careful. Notably, emotional intelligence is distinct from I.Q., on which both John and Harry would probably score, by their planning and abstract decision-making, very highly.

Disclaimer: The views about places, events, and automobile types do not necessarily reflect the author's opinions, and some aspects have been overemphasized to add color to the tale.

Restoration I

The Power of Nutrition

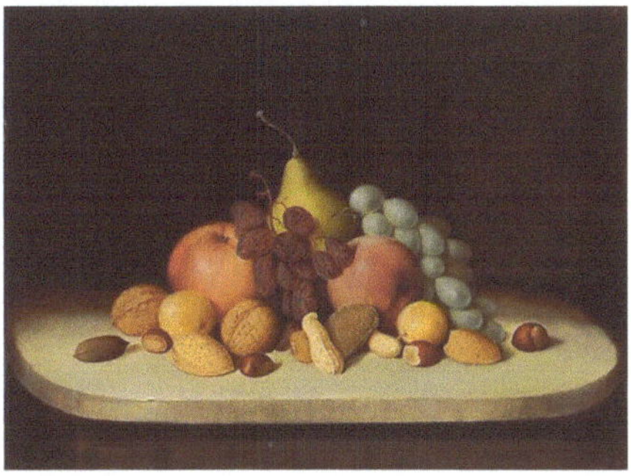

The image above is: Still life with fruits and nuts painted by the artist Robert Seldon Duncanson (1848).

Classically composed of fruit arranged in a tabletop pyramid, the painting includes remarkable passages juxtaposing the smooth surfaces of beautifully rendered apples with the textured shells of scattered nuts. This painting reflects on this chapter's main message that perhaps the most important brain foods come from fruits, nuts, and their respective oils.

This chapter proposes a balanced diet for brain health, which emphasizes an omnivorous diet.

John was having a nightmare.

A horrible nightmare. The kind of nightmare that you awaken from with a vivid memory of all that transpired, only to forget it in the morning. John had learned not to try to remember. In any case, he knew nightmares had no connection with reality, but were an echo of some kind of unresolved stress that had not been dealt with in the conscious state. John knew that many cultures believed in a dream world, and also that this could become nightmarish. In that world, it was possible to make changes and to re-enter that nightmare to fix what went wrong. However possible that was, he knew one could not 'fix' the stress from which it emanated. That stress was the Gordian knot, which, when unraveled, was the progenitor to all sorts of behaviors that did not really work well to resolve the problem. One of these behaviors was drinking too much, while others include using substances to "forget"; or habitually taking chances at a gambling casino (where all the odds are stacked against you). The oblivion of randomness was one solution. John knew that the illogical could appear to become the solution to the logic of 'stress' and all that can emanate from it.

In that world of stress, nothing makes too much sense. Time becomes a commodity that can, seemingly, be bought by the advancement of technology and the emergence of more electronics...or so some people seem to think. It goes like this: by shrinking the world, everything becomes more crowded, and one becomes one's own avatar. Pretty shocking!

This "fix it" world usually has an answer for the physical

world. In a nutshell, the physical body is a temple, and you have to shape it to become what you want. With that ultimate control - to change who you are, or worse, hide who you really are - you can change the way you feel. Indeed, this emphasis on the physical form also stems from the belief that the way you look can modify the way you feel about yourself.

John found all this to be partially true, but there was a flaw at the heart of the argument, in much the same way there was a flaw in the argument for the duality of mind and body; in the real sense, they are a united whole.

So, John pondered, *why do people wake up in the morning to go for a run to tone their bodies, but no one seems to wake up to take their brain for a run?*

Surely, a well-exercised brain can also affect the body? And, what about giving the brain the right food to solve the problems of the body and mind? Better still, why not look at it from the other side? John's reasoning was as follows: accelerate physical health to "tone the brain" and eat the right foods to "feed the brain"; in turn, these will fine-tune the body as well. Taken to its logical conclusion, the right foods and the right amount of physical exercise can "tone the brain" and be a solution for stress, as well as all that it can give rise to, including; drinking and drugging to excess, and taking all those unneeded (note that the word 'unnecessary' was not used) risks.

Why not go a step further, John thought?

Is there a general theory that can bring all these together, which ancient humans knew instinctively, but is now mostly forgotten? What are our powers to "restore" our brains? Can foods and exercise reverse the scourge of stress, so we can regain control over excessive indulgence in drink, drugs, and all those other behaviors we would rather avoid? Is there really a "gut feeling" that affects our brain's functionality? John needed to talk with his friend Astronuff. Now, he was a real genius and seemed to have an easy way to understand everything. Why not make this even more fun and bring a few students along?

The Silent Organ

John had known Astronuff since his time at Oxford. Astronuff was one of those people you would easily pass by on the street, thinking he had just escaped from a homeless shelter. Astronuff was not just scruffy; he was downright unkempt. His favorite attire was a seemingly moth-eaten sweater and what seemed to be a converted, wet, sheepskin rug. His beard was untamed, and you would never find him without a lit cigarette in his mouth. How on earth could this man be a genius? Well, the world works in mysterious ways! And so did Astronuff.

Astronuff was a Viking. His primary goal was to have as many kids as possible who were boys. He loved recounting Viking crusades even though he purported to be a Christian, and alluded to being nothing more complicated than that! He did not believe in publishing his ideas, because that was too neo-classical a concept. In his view, the only time one ought to publish anything was when it could change the world. And, he was too modest to think that any of his ideas would do that.

His most intriguing idea at Oxford, where he and John had shared a small office, was that he could get a PC/MAC to have the processing power of a small part of a lizard's brain. This was way before the age of supercomputers. Undaunted by his lack of programming skills, Astronuff learned C Programming in just three days, and C++ in only about two weeks, practically becoming an expert programmer. This usually took years! Intrigued, John had helped him to build what would now be seen as primitive neural (machine learning) networks to give some "intelligence" to his programming. No one dared to argue with Astronuff, except John, for fear that he harbored ideas that would win at least a couple of Noble prizes, which everyone else was too dumb to understand. This cerebral sparring with his then-colleague was challenging, but John had the moxie to do it as he feared no other intellect. John's strongest belief was that he could understand anything that had a reasonable explanation. This was going to be fun!

John reached out to Astronuff when he was due to give a few lectures at Oxford as part of his summer vacation.

"Hello Astronuff, this is John," the caller explained over the phone. "Fancy a pint of beer while I am at Oxford next week?"

"Certainly, John," Astronuff replied. "But knowing you, it will be several beers.

"Okay if I bring Pamela along?" he added, not expecting much of a reply.

"With pleasure," said John. "Will 6 pm at the Eagle and Child do?"

Astronuff knew the implications of that statement. This had been a famous meeting place for literary geniuses like C.S. Lewis and J.R. Tolkien. "Splendid," he finally answered.

"You are veering off the beaten path, aren't you?" Astronuff added a couple of beats later.

"Till then," John dismissed.

He became uneasy and somewhat nervous. On the set day, John arrived first, found himself a prime corner, and sat nursing a pint of Guinness. Astronuff had not changed one bit in the last decade. Pamela, the woman accompanying him, was a surprise, though.

She was a youngish girl with vibrant red hair and a nose clip - not much like a Ph.D. student, John thought. Still, looks could be deceiving. And so they proved to be as soon as they sat down. Pamela was a Rhodes scholar and sharper than a straight edge. Physically, she was a striking contrast to Astronuff, who could well have blurred into the background.

Astronuff got himself a pint of Bass pale ale and the same for Pamela, who was hard to miss on account of her constant hair-tossing. Astronuff started to puff on a smokeless vape; regular smoking had been banned in British pubs more than a decade earlier.

"What's on your mind, John? I brought Pamela - a member of the new wave of radical thinking in science - along to assist. Not many of those left. Science is dying, John. Stuffed with self-important committees extolling the little we actually know. There is more dialog in a monastery...and certainly a lot more beer!" stated Astronuff, who was definitely not in good form tonight.

"Astronuff, let's make this simple. Why do people not take their brains seriously? Why do they not think or believe that the brain has dominion over all the body?" asked John.

"Sounds like you paraphrased a line out of Milton's Paradise Lost, not real science, just fantasy," Astronuff responded. "There are no dominions in the body - just components. Many so critical for continuous immediate survival, and having only one exist for each. If you were an engineer in charge of manufacturing humans, would you not have designed the most critical organs to have duplicates?"

Here Pamela joined in.

"And the single most important, the brain, appears to be the most exposed; and a greedy organ at that too, consuming about 20% of the body's energy resources. No one would ever design an Android like a human; just wouldn't make any sense."

Astronuff continued, "Most people treat their brains as though they are redundant. It is one of the SILENT ORGANS! People think that if you cannot feel it, it is not important. We think our hearts are important because we can feel them beating. And when we were very young children, we could even hear it beating. No one ever heard their brain working, so no one takes their brain seriously. Just like no one takes their liver seriously as they cannot feel it work. So, the only time we think about any silent organ is when it is so diseased, we cannot help but notice the incapacity. The same goes for the liver, by the way. So, John, that answer is easy."

"We do not think our brains to be important because we cannot truly perceive them working," concluded Pamela. She went on, "It's even worse than that because the other so-called silent organs are not truly silent, but they "whisper". For instance, we know our kidneys are working because we urinate, and we know our liver and bowels are working because we have to use the restroom to excrete fecal waste. The brain - considering its substantial size, positioning, and power drainage - really is the silent one. Yes, we know that there are small internal organs we do not ever hear of, like the pancreas, but they are not the size or dominance of the brain, although they do make their presence felt in disease, just like the brain".

"Wow. I hadn't really thought of it that way," John reflected. "If only we could make our brains be heard in some way, perhaps then we would be inspired to keep it in top shape? Could it be that simple?"

Oxidative Stress

"Do you think they will let us into the famous 'Rabbit Room'?" Astronuff quipped.

"I do not know. It's usually for the top literary boffins, isn't it? It's where C.S. Lewis and his buddies met. It would have been great to have heard all those burgeoning stories, though," said John. "Wish they were scientists," he continued after a moment, "they might have had stories closer to what we are mulling over now."

"Wrong city," Pamela interrupted their wishful thinking. "That would be at the 'other place'; the second-best University in the UK, not here."

"Oh, stop that. My cousin was a professor there, and he was no dunce. Besides, they have more Nobel Laureates in science than we do! So perhaps, it's we who are in the wrong place. What do we know about literature?" John responded with an unusual flash of irritation. "And besides, quite a good deal of what I want to talk about came from there."

There was a lull in conversation as everyone had their drinks refilled.

"Well, if we're all ready now, here is the other issue; I think the brain talks to us when it is stressed. Everyone is used to their muscles being stressed and aching, that's easy, but the brain being stressed leads to all sorts of poor outcomes too. The key principle here is what is called 'oxidative stress'. The most vulnerable people are not even aware that this phenomenon exists," Astronuff opened.

"How does that truly manifest?" asked John.

Pamela stood up like a shot, pointing to some invisible blackboard.

"Oxidative stress is an imbalance between free radicals and antioxidants in the body. Free radicals are molecules that carry oxygen with an uneven number of electrons. They cause a large number of complicated chain reactions in the body and react with almost every other molecule that they come across, causing oxidation. Sometimes, this is good, but mostly, it is bad. Now, here is how antioxidants come into play: You remember that the free radicals have an uneven number of electrons? Well, the antioxidants donate electrons to them, without becoming unstable themselves, making an even number of electrons that are now not so reactive. Antioxidants are really good for you in general and great for your brain. Now, many people confuse the oxygen, which we breathe, with oxidation. They are not the same thing. But I will not digress."

Catching her breath, Pamela continued. "Oxidative stress can lead to you becoming ill with high blood pressure, hardening of your arteries (atherosclerosis), diabetes, and the likes. Most importantly, it leads to a degeneration of your brain. It may even explain why we get diseases such as Parkinson's and Alzheimer's. Drinking too much alcohol, taking drugs, smoking, or even overeating are real brain killers! Oxidative stress happens to be why we die...but that's a story I can tell later. The great thing here, boys, is that if we eat the right things, we can reduce this oxidative stress. Not through the easy way - popping vitamins which are thought to have antioxidant properties - but through eating real food, real food for real people. Food devoid of props intended to make pharmaceutical companies money."

"That is all well," said John, "but do you know that the burning matter on my mind is how oxidative stress relates to consuming an excess of alcohol? Now, let me tell you some of what I know."

Oxidative Stress And Alcohol Consumption

John got ready. It was now his time to be the "Professor".

"I know you think too much reading is a bit recherché, Astronuff, but I did read this fascinating article by a chap called Wu."

"Who?" asked Astronuff in confusion.

"Wu. Defeng Wu, not 'who'," clarified John. "Wu describes these highly-reactive oxygen molecules, let's call them the Reactive Oxygen Species (ROS), that are quite destructive to many reactions within the cells of our body. Alcohol promotes the conversion of xanthine dehydrogenase to xanthine oxidase (Sultatos, 1988), which generates these ROS molecules, and these, in turn, enhance oxidative stress. Without being checked by antioxidants, oxidative stress associated with alcohol use:

Causes spiral reactions in the NAD+/NADPH ratio which interfere with the breakdown of alcohol, increase acetaldehyde in the cell, thereby creating even further damage, promoting even more ROS;

Damages mitochondria - the intracellular organelles that produce energy within the cell - and, in so doing, starve the cells of oxygen. This is a process known as cellular hypoxia;

Tells our immune system to start producing cytokines (basically signaling an immune war against an unknown agent), thus allowing endotoxins produced by bacteria to enter the cells and hide; and

Causes its own vicious cycle of destruction by unbinding metals from proteins, and producing its own radical, called the 1-hydroxyethyl radical. Not only is this harmful to your brain cells, but it is also really bad for liver cells because it affects the ability of P450 molecules to break down products. Hence, you would be unable to break down toxins in your food efficiently (and this is actually a vital process in the production of alcohol-induced liver damage).

"While there is some relief due to the transient production of CYP2E1 (Lieber, 1977) to metabolize alcohol, this is, itself, overwhelmed by excessive alcohol consumption."

Realizing he had essentially monopolized the conversation, John decided to check he still had an audience.

"Would you like to know more?"

"Don't let us stop your lecture," Pamela responded, gesturing for him to go on.

"Matter of fact, I wish I was taking some notes."

"Just like John," Astronuff huffed, "to be a bloody encyclopedia."

John, however, was undeterred.

"What's worse is that people do not know what's right for

them and so take supplements like crazy, without knowing quite what they are doing. Remember that I said that alcohol consumption frees iron from proteins in the cell? Well, guess what? If you drink too much, you will have a situation where your cells are overloaded with iron. And if you simply give everyone who drinks excessively some more iron, because you heard someone who drinks too much might have anemia, then voila, you have another thing coming! Your liver cannot handle all this iron, and you would end up with liver damage (Sadrzadeh et al. 1994; Tsukamoto et al. 1995; Nanji and Hiller-Sturmhöfel 1997). All these have been known for decades! To make matters worse, all this ROS activity can damage your DNA, leading to all sorts of mutations and cancers. Canadians are smart. They have warning labels on alcoholic beverages stating they can cause cancer - why is this not done everywhere?"

"And," John sailed on, "here is what you can do to really ramp up the vicious cycle of damage caused by oxidative stress: increase your levels of natural radiation by sitting in the sun and absorbing excessive amounts of UV light; sit around in a smog infested city, rather than being outdoors or by the seaside, or countryside; smoke or inhale secondary smoke; and yes, even just stress your body out or get too little sleep. All these are recipes for early death."

"I do not feel like drinking anymore," said Pamela. "You've really ruined the night. I thought this was meant to be a little fun with two old professors. Instead, you tell me I am sitting with you chaps drinking poison."

"Steady on," said John, "although alcohol can cause these

effects, there are many natural processes to reduce the damage. I will get there in a minute if you let me."

"You'd better get on with it quickly. You seem to have drawn quite a crowd," Astronuff scoffed. Sure enough, little groups had gathered around their table. "We risk being thrown out of this place, never to return, if everyone stops drinking. You really should keep your voice down a bit when you get excited, professor," he scolded.

Combating Oxidative Stress Through General Behaviors And Nutrition

John shuffled in his chair, but then, decided to get up, as he could feel eyes like daggers in his back anyway.

"I-I wrote a small side paper on this some time ago but did not get many thanks... except from one really nice chap. His recipe, (now expanded to 15 items) may make you smarter, and perhaps, even help you curb your drinking too much. It will certainly reduce the damage alcohol use can do to your brain and the rest of your body, and can check the habit of eating a lot of the wrong foods. I also recommend certain ways of living, or should I say being, which I wish I followed myself as I would certainly feel much better.

"In a concise summary, here goes:

General Behaviors

These are some things we all really can do at least some of:

Do not sit in the sun or spend too much time out in it. If you must go out in the sun, wear sunscreen - no matter your skin color or complexion;

Use cleaning chemicals with caution; they are buzzing with free radicals trying to latch on to all that dirt;

Sleep well. Your body requires adequate sleep to produce antioxidants;

Try to avoid over-eating, which puts your body in a state of constant oxidative stress; and

Exercise moderately and regularly to increase your body's level of antioxidants (especially aerobic exercise). This will also slow down your aging, keep you healthier, and make you live longer. Later in this book, there is more on what constitutes "adequate" aerobic exercise.

Nutrition - now let us put some of that biochemistry to use:

a). Supplements. You may recall that I cautioned about taking excessive iron and iron supplements if you drink too much because that can lead to further damage. But, there are certain supplements you really should pay some attention to. But first, just a little more biochemistry; there's a system in the body called the glutathione peroxidase system. It includes multiple components like the enzyme glutathione peroxidase, glutathione reductase, the cofactor glutathione, and reduced levels of Nicotinamide Adenosine Dinucleotide Phosphate (NADPH).

ROS molecules are removed from the body by superoxide dismutases, which clear out the superoxide radicals. Critical to the efficient working of this ROS protection system is a group of elements that are needed and should be present at low levels in the cell. These include selenium, manganese, copper, and zinc. Note that an oversupply of these supplements will provide no added benefits and might even be harmful to the liver. So, the first recommendation is to ensure adequate levels of selenium, manganese, copper, and zinc in the body. This can be achieved through a balanced diet. If this is not possible due to bowel disease or nutritional choices, the use of appropriate supplements under medical supervision will also do the trick.

The second set of recommendations would be to ensure the intake of B vitamins and Thiamin, which are important co-factors for brain metabolism and neuronal health. Vitamins A, D, E, and K are also important supplements if you are not getting them from your diet as their intake can be inhibited by excessive alcohol consumption. Other smart choices would be glutathione as an antioxidant, and vitamin C to help bolster the immune system.

b) Blueberries can help protect the brain from oxidative stress, which can reduce the symptoms of age-related mental conditions like Alzheimer's and other forms of dementia.

c) Nuts and seeds of all varieties are high in vitamin E and, as a result, help resist cognitive decline. You could regularly eat nuts like Brazil nuts, peanuts, flaxseed, almonds, and sunflower seeds.

d) Whole grains can help you lose weight and make you physically fit. They also help to prevent heart disease, which eventually ensures your brain is working smarter.

e) Dark chocolate, due to its powerful antioxidant properties, can help enhance your focus and improve your concentration. Half an ounce of this a day is sufficient.

f) Freshly brewed tea that is not powdered or bottled. Taking as much as two to three cups a day will offer your brain a modest amount of caffeine, which will help you to focus and concentrate better. Powdered or bottled teas should be avoided since they are usually less effective.

g) Avocados have similar properties to blueberries and

also promote healthy blood flow in your body, and especially to your brain, because of the good fat in them.

h) Wild salmon and other deepwater fishes help improve your brain performance due to the high amount of omega-3 fatty acids in them. Indeed, Omega-3 fatty acids are critical for overall brain health. They are polyunsaturated fats, containing essential products like eicosapentaenoic acid (EPA) and docosahexaenoic acid (DPA). EPA and DPA are so critical to brain function that their levels in pregnancy are correlated with higher scores on intelligence tests (Helland B et al., 2003; Oken et al. 2005) conducted on offspring, and can reduce cognitive decline in adults (Yurko-Mauro et al., 2020).

John recalled that as a child, his father always had his sister and him take a capsule of cod liver oil for years! At the time, John did not like to take such "yukky" things, but he grew to love - to that day - wild salmon. In older adults, decreased levels of DPA are associated with reduced brain size.

"Do not overdo it, though," John continued. "The US FDA has set a safe upper limit for the intake of omega-3 fatty acid supplements as 3000 mg a day, whilst the European Food and Safety Authority has placed their recommended maximum dose higher at 5,000 mg a day. Now, getting back to the list. Where was I? Finished the eighth, I believe?

i) Beans will help you stabilize your level of blood sugar, resulting in better performance for your brain.

j) Pomegranate juice, whether drunk as juice or taken from the fruit, has been shown through research to have better antioxidant benefits than red wine and green tea, which is good news since that means taking pomegranate can help your brain function better.

k) Beets, due to the fact that they are rich in vitamin B, will ensure, when regularly consumed, the abundance of the nutrients that will help you process data and sort through memories quickly. Make sure to avoid canned beets, though.

l) Eggs are also rich in omega-3 fatty acids that will protect your brain. Taking eggs regularly can help make you "smarter", as well as prevent diseases like Alzheimer's.

m) Spinach is rich in iron, which helps prevent brain development problems in infants and adults. Be careful of excessive ingestion of iron if you consume a lot of alcohol.

n) Kale has anti-aging agents that lowers the age of your brain, thereby making it function more effectively.

o) Apples contain substances that protect you from brain-damaging chemicals. It is important to only eat organic apples, though, since these substances are in the fruit's skin."

There are additional foods that have known anti-inflammatory properties. For example, salmon contains omega-3-fatty acids, which when served roasted, poached, or steamed can help reduce inflammation. Spices such as tumeric also have anti-inflammatory properties and when combined with black pepper is better absorbed. Flax seeds, chai seeds, and granola are important for a balanced anti-inflammation diet, and adding walnuts to salads can serve to improve flavor to food items such as salads as well as improve its anti-inflammatory properties. Above all, drink lots of water!

John rounded up his comment with a flourish.

"You do know that there are foods you should try and avoid

if you drink too much, right? Basically, anything that leads to a rapid intake of excessive sugar. This can be fatal if your brain is starved of certain molecules called co-factors, which drive a biological process called the Krebs cycle. If the Krebs cycle is impaired, there is inefficient handling of cellular respiration. In short, there is a shortage of hydrogen and electrons to drive the energy organelles in the brain; the mitochondria. This leads to an uncontrolled amount of sugar in the brain, which is broken down into an abundance of ketones. This "charge" of ketones and sugar in the brain can send you into a coma or even kill you. I suppose that will be that then!" John completed.

The small audience in the pub did not know exactly what they were witnessing, but it was all a bit amusing. An odder group of people than you would ever think could be acquainted with one another were here in one place, talking about science and food at the same time. This could happen in a few places other than Oxford, which was full of really clever people hanging about, seemingly not doing much. The audience was too sophisticated to ask for a calling card from the participants as the anonymity of the group conveyed its own credibility. And why would anyone even clap? This was just regular pub banter amongst colleagues.

John was exhausted and dumped himself back in his seat. Pamela had whipped out her cell phone to make sure the babysitter had not left, and Astronuff was stroking his beard, making it uglier-looking in the diffused lighting of the pub.

"Not sure what more to say, John. Your list of foods allows, by my calculation, for over one trillion different recipes -

perhaps much more. Which is more than enough to eat through in a lifetime, so it can be done," said Astronuff.

Typical of Astronuff. He had reduced this all to a math equation of primes, thought John.

"Time to call it a day, Astronuff and Pamela?" he asked.

"I suppose so" came the collective reply, and they all gathered their coats and grudgingly made for the door. It seemed like the night was somewhat incomplete, but the next steps were less certain. No one seemed to be in the mood for more booze, or a quick sprint to the kebab house for a late-night snack. More reflection was needed.

"Cheers," shouted John as they spilled into the street. He, too, knew this was to be continued...but where? By whom? And how?

Signature Appendix: Oxford Notes

The Eagle and Child is best known as the meeting place of the Inklings - an informal literary group that included C.S. Lewis and J.R.R Tolkien. A plaque in a corner that was part of the 'Rabbit Room' commemorates where they met regularly. Apparently, this pub also served as the lodgings of the Chancellor of the Exchequer during the Civil War.

The Krebs Cycle

The diagram below shows how this part of respiration is an ever-repeating cycle that produces ATP and gives off carbon dioxide (CO_2). The Adenosine Triphosphate (ATP) is a molecule which carries energy in chemical form to be used in other cell processes. To summarize:

Two molecules of carbon dioxide are given off

One molecule of Guanosine Triphosphate (GTP) is formed

Three molecules of Nicotinamide adenine dinucleotide (NAD+) are combined with hydrogen (NAD+ → NADH)

One molecule of Flavin Adenine Dinucleotide (FAD) combines with hydrogen (FAD → $FADH_2$)

Because two acetyl-CoA molecules are produced from each glucose molecule, two cycles are required per glucose molecule. Therefore, at the end of two cycles, the products are: two ATP, six NADH, two FADH2, two QH2 (ubiquinol), and four CO2.

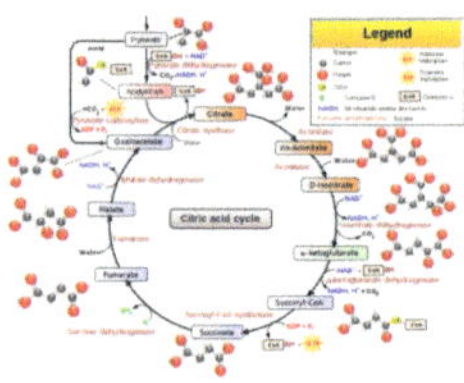

The diagram above is: The citric acid cycle (Krebs cycle) - simplified overview.

See Also

What's the difference between NAD+ and NADH?

What's the difference between FAD and NADH

Restoration II

An Application Of Nutrition

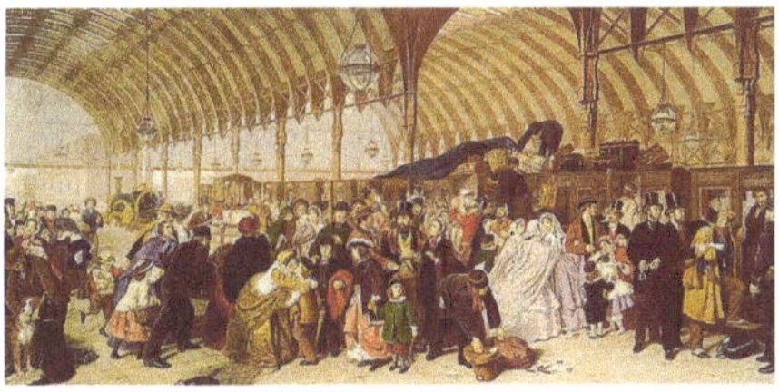

The image above is: The Railway Station (1862) - William Powell Frith.

William Powell Frith (1819-1909) was one of the greatest portrayers of nineteenth-century life. The featured painting is Frith's The Railway Station (Royal Holloway College). It was set in London's Paddington Station, completed a decade before, built by the great Victorian engineer Isambard Kingdom Brunel. Paddington was a cutting-edge building, constructed from cast iron and glass, and at the time, lit by gaslight.

It was a beautiful - no - a simply gorgeous day in Oxford. John relished the taxi drive across the bridge spanning the river Cherwell and past the Magdalen Tower. He remembered, most fondly, standing at the bottom of the tower at 6 AM on May Morning to listen to what sounded like a most angelic choir singing *Hymnus Eucharisticus*, a tradition dating back to Henry VII, some 500 years ago. But this was not a frosty May Morning, it was the middle of summer, and the spires of the Magdalen tower could be seen for miles.

It was not the fastest route to the Medical Research Council Unit at Oxford University in the Warneford Hospital, where he had agreed to meet Astronuff and Pamela again. John was running exactly 4 minutes late, but he believed that time was the ultimate luxury, and to spend a few extra minutes of it the way you wanted was simply heaven on earth.

John was looking forward to seeing Astronuff again, and of course, Pamela. It had been several months since their wintery discussion at the Eagle and Child pub, and for John, some of the ideas had begun to settle in his head. Today's quest was to understand the application of nutrition to brain health, particularly to support those with excessive drinking habits, or those whose use of substances had gotten out of their control.

John knew his way around well at the Medical Research Council Unit (MRC) - not many years ago, he too had been bustling down the same halls.

Was I ever that young? he wondered, as he brushed past students.

Astronuff's room was right at the end of the hall on the first plan. He liked this perch, as he could sit on the window ledge and sneak a quick fag. How could any doctor nowadays smoke?

But Astronuff was from a truly bygone era, and it was best to accept him as he presented himself. Pamela was already in her colleague's office when the guest arrived. She looked strangely different today; certainly prettier with her long hair tied up neatly in a knot at the back. The nose ring was nowhere to be seen. It took all of John's resolve not to ask Pamela what she had done with it. Now, that would have been politically incorrect, perhaps on any day, let alone at Oxford in the present day.

Astronuff wasn't interested in talking about nutrition. Instead, he was embroiled in a discussion about how distracted everyone in the world was, and how no one did any real thinking anymore. Indeed, he didn't care much about nutrition; his philosophy was simply to eat until his stomach hurt. Even though he was a brilliant scientist and knew that the brain received signals from the stomach and that it took several full minutes before the effects could be consciously realized, he did not seem cautioned to eat more slowly. In fact, it didn't seem to matter to him at all. It was simply his philosophy of life - indulge as much as possible for as long as you could get away with it.

Astronuff rose to greet John with a huge hug, as if they had not seen each other for several years. Pamela, keeping her distance, reached out with an outstretched hand.

"Good trip up from London?" Astronuff asked.

John had practically forgotten his trip on the train from London to Oxford station, as that had been blurred by such a wondrous taxi ride from the station to the MRC Unit. How true was Astronuff's observation about how utterly distracted the world had become?

"Astronuff," began John, "I had a strange encounter on the train with some lost soul."

"Tell us about it," chirped Pamela, as she poured some Earl Grey tea into their teacups and passed around a few, rather damp, biscuits.

"Sure thing," said John.

Here is how John's train journey from Paddington station in London to Oxford passed.

The Train Journey

The two men, John and Samuel, met as if by accident on a train ride; each headed to his individual destination, but also, having very different feelings about how the day would transpire.

John, a doctor by training, was a man who had gone to all the right schools but had fewer years left ahead than behind. He had a keen comportment that flattered his years and was feeling optimistic about the day. John was a man of minute observational precision, just the sort who still wore a mechanical watch, calibrated perfectly to time. Yes, John revered *Patek Phillipe* as a brand, but not for a trip like what lay ahead. On that day, John's choice was a *Louis Moinet Memoris*, a brand invented by the maker of the first chronograph. A watch that told a story, but was not ostentatious by name or appearance as to instantly draw much attention of anyone, but a connoisseur. He was headed to Oxford to give a talk, not for a social gathering. John would never indulge in the casual laziness of an electronic watch, although few people had greater computerized sophistication.

John was always no more than 6 minutes late, never more, never less; the time it took to be noticed, but not be stared at.

Samuel was about two decades younger. For his part, he had sort of done the right things, almost went to all the right schools, but was a great success nonetheless. He was an adopter of the 'modern age', trusting all his knowledge to what he read online and considered libraries to be not much different from museums. Samuel was wealthy, accomplished, and an astute businessman, with the canny skill of being able to "read" the person in front of him.

John and Samuel's initial contact had been one of painful awkwardness. Samuel had sat next to John and whipped out his cellular phone - no signal. He shuffled uncomfortably to reach for his other phone in his briefcase, yet there was still no signal! Samuel looked beyond himself just long enough to catch John's wry smile as he muttered, "Welcome to our undistracted new planet."

Samuel had met John's type before...or so he thought. Obviously, a bored, middle-aged man without much to do, just looking to pick a fight with someone. He ignored him.

John was not, however, ready to give up on the encounter and tried again.

"Going home to be with the family"?

"No, just off to a meeting," came Samuel's clipped reply. "I can never tell why the network seldom works on these trains. Just frustrating!" he followed up.

"Well, perhaps, we can talk," said John.

Samuel shrugged.

Taking this as his cue, John continued. "My name is John."

Samuel replied, "Just call me Sam."

"I'll call you Samuel," replied John.

The owner of the name shrugged again.

"Did you happen to notice how many people are sat behind you, Samuel?"

Samuel was puzzled.

What kind of a quiz is this? he wondered. *Am I being filmed?*

"Six!" John said quickly.

"How did you guess?" asked "Sam."

"Well, I counted. You never know when such a thing might come in useful. I also noticed the color of their shoes. The lady sitting at the end of the row was most noticeable with her bright red shoe with blue socks," said John.

"Do you do this for a living?" enquired an even more puzzled Samuel. "Like, some sort of gambler or card player?"

"Nothing of the sort," replied John, "I'm just a country doctor. I was born into a world that, most likely, sounds like science fiction to you. There were no cell phones until I was what I would presume to be your age, and even those were the size of a small suitcase. Yes, and computers were the size of a room."

"You must be 100 years old!" Samuel stated.

"Feels like that, but in reality, I was perhaps just that much older than you are now at the turn of the millennium. Won't see the next one though, but neither will you nor anyone else on this train," John said, muttering the last line.

Samuel had now gained back some of his composure and realized that he had never quite met someone like John. He was not annoying, but strangely fascinating just by being a little bit offbeat at times. Samuel was curious.

"Tell me more about the lady's shoe and why that could ever be important to notice," Samuel asked John.

John began, "Because it was all most fascinating. Let me explain: Six reminds me of a hexagon - most perfect shape in nature - and the red shoe, being amongst all the other black ones worn by other people, introduced an asymmetry into the form. Asymmetries are important to observe because they can denote change, and since she happened to be dressed rather oddly and sitting next to the fire extinguisher, I thought it was worth just one more glance. As to the importance, I could not very well tell you for sure, but it did cross my mind that she had the red shoe on her artificial foot, and should we need that fire extinguisher, we could be in a bit of a pickle."

"Well, I am a financier in the City, and I do not much believe in a string of coincidences, let alone spending this much time working out every nuance of every chance encounter. Just too busy. I am sure a call would have come into my phone before I even had time to notice anyone," said Samuel. "In any case, the observation is useless, we will never need the fire extinguisher, and it would not have mattered if there were up to 7 people sitting behind us. Quite irrelevant!"

John smiled kindly at Samuel and continued. "Perhaps not so irrelevant for your brain. Multiple possibilities do add up to a probability in a lifetime. However, in the last 10 minutes, something marvelous occurred. Your brain was tasked with focus, recall of pictorial memory, a little math, associative analysis, risk assessment, and perhaps, above all that, you made a new friend. Better than being distracted by that phone, which, I hope, our conversation allowed you to withdraw from. If you can do something like this for just 2 minutes of each hour, your mind, more precisely, your brain, will always be in top condition for the next meeting. No need for coffee; just use your brain to create its own stimulation."

"Are you for real?" asked Samuel.

"Quite so," John replied. He continued, "Now, I know the situation of the people behind us was sort of strange, but I do try and notice the world around me. Saved me from many a car accident. While driving, once I notice that the person behind me is on his cell phone, I reduce my speed and brake slowly, allowing him to catch up in time. To that driver, the dangerous myth of multitasking was being effected. Simply put, it does not really exist. We cannot really multitask as we do not have multi-phase brains. But, like I said, thinking about these things seems to keep me out of trouble."

"Were you not a strange one at school - teased or bullied?" Samuel asked of John.

The other replied, "Well, I was lucky...I did not quite go to a school like that. Here, there is an allegorical tale I would like to tell you. Nothing to do with me. Basically, the bottom line is: do not get distracted by the distracter. The tale goes like this:

A young man walks into an interview to gain entrance into an esteemed college. The interviewer is reading a newspaper when the man comes in and asks him to sit. The young man decides not to disturb the interviewer - more polite that way, he thinks! Ten minutes later, the interviewer looks up and tells the young man that he can leave.

'How did I do?' asks the young man.

'Well, seeing as you never said a word, not well.'

The young man replied indignantly, 'How can you say that when you were reading a newspaper?'

'Ah,' the interviewer replied, 'I did that to see if I could distract you. It worked. You should have valued your time and removed the newspaper from my hand. Then, I would have known we were on the same plane of reference. By sitting there and being silent, you allowed yourself to be in an alien world without protest and identified with an alienist. Perhaps this school is not for you.'"

"By the way," said John, as his tale ended, "We are heading towards the home of one of the greatest schools on earth."

The train stopped at the station at the end of the terminal, and everyone began to get their luggage.

"My cell batteries just died! What time is it?" asked Samuel.

"I do not really know," John replied as he looked at his watch, "but it looks as if we're perfectly 2 minutes late on arrival. And do tie up those shoelaces, so you do not fall over."

The Meeting

Pamela's eyes brightened, and with a flashing smile, she asked, "John was that a true story?"

"As true as we are actually here," replied John.

Pamela knew his implication. You had to be on the same plane of thought to make comments about the characters in the story.

John continued, "I bet Samuel, when he woke up this morning, did not at all think of what he would eat or drink to optimize his brain."

At this, Astronuff looked up. "Brain food? You mean like coffee?"

"No. Not quite," John answered.

A few years earlier, John had come up with the idea to create some beverages to optimize the brain. It had been a creation out of necessity; his pregnant wife had asked him to go to the grocery store to buy her favorite vitamin-infused beverage. Arriving at the store, and reaching into a shelf to read the label on the back of the bottles, he was aghast at what he saw. The vitamin drinks contained hardly *any* vitamins, and certainly not enough to do much of any good for anyone. To make matters worse, these drinks were all heavily laced with sugar and caffeine to deliver an instant jolt, only to bring the consumer crashing back to earth a short while later. These alternations of highs and lows would create their own "addiction", a yearning for the rush - and the consumer would get hooked. John called to complain to his wife that these drinks would not be good for her.

She had responded with a professorial sounding voice, "Then go and invent something better."

What a challenge! John had thought. Then, a few short weeks later, *voila!*, he had mixed up a set of drinks that were not saturated with sugar or caffeine, and had a chance to actually stimulate the brain. A true brain drink, if you like. This had not been as easy as it sounded.

The brain is not a gland!

It's not as simple as noting a deficiency which is rare in a healthy brain and simply providing nutrients to replenish what is lacking. For example, the thyroid is a gland. If there are low levels of thyroid hormone, you can simply give a supplement, levothyroxine, to raise thyroid hormone levels. The brain, however, works in a very different way. It is not possible to access the brain simply and directly. The brain protects itself through a blood-barrier so it is not bombarded by toxic chemicals. The organ is quite selective about what it lets into itself. Getting these vitamins and nutrients accepted required that the drinks be balanced and have the right concentrations. To be even more granular, choices had to be made about which ingredients were chosen from the wide variety, which, in turn, depended on finding the 'right' atomic weight and structure.

"Wow!" Pamela exclaimed at this information. "Did you really spend only a few weeks on this?"

Comfortable that he now had their attention, John answered, "Afraid so."

Of course, John knew this was an exercise in theoretical knowledge, as he had not actually run clinical trials to prove his ideas, but, in his defense, there was quite a lot of good science about the ingredients individually. The clinical trials, if needed (and to whoever did run clinical trials on soft drinks), would have to come later. John was not "claiming" anything but his ideas, and people could choose to drink or disregard it as they pleased. At the time, he was simply blending a recipe to tackle a curious problem posed by his wife. But now that he had turned his mind to it, why not flesh out a few added beverages to embrace the challenge fully? John knew these tonics had to aid not just those in good health, but also, those who might be over-indulging in alcohol and other substances, or whose behavioral needs were otherwise not being met.

He provided a brief synopsis of the beverages he had come up with:

INSPIRE™ was conceptualized on the principal that

thiamine is essential for the nervous system and can be reduced by excessive alcohol intake, leading to neurological disease. Thiamine could alleviate, or perhaps, prevent hangovers by supplying co-factors for the Krebs Cycle (See chapter entitled Restoration - I). Riboflavin is an essential nutrient required for numerous cellular processes, including the balance of monoamines in the brain. Niacin increases blood flow to the brain. Vitamin B-12 & B-6 can help reduce drowsiness and promote mental alertness, along with helping to create hemoglobin, which carries oxygen to the brain. Biotin is a metabolic transmitter known to have a detoxifying effect, and can help combat lethargy. Magnesium can calm the nervous system. Notably, INSPIRE™ contains citicoline and a small amount of caffeine, which, in a randomized placebo-controlled double-blind study of 60 healthy participants, was shown to lead to "significantly faster maze learning times and reaction times on a continuous performance test, fewer errors in a go/no-go task and better accuracy on a measure of information processing speed", and improved P450 EEG amplitude that "indicates a general improvement in the ability to accommodate new and relevant information within working memory, and overall enhanced brain activation" (Bruce et al.,2014).. Finally, citicoline appears to be important in humans to improve working memory and, in Europe, is used as part of a treatment for Alzheimer's disease, Parkinson's disease, and memory loss. John further theorized that INSPIRE™ would not only be an interesting brain food to enhance brain activity, acuity, and sharpness, but could also comprise a strategy to help individuals suffering hangovers, as its osmotic capabilities could aid cellular hydration.

HAPPY™ was blended to enhance moods, tranquility, bliss, and a sense of well-being. Niacin helps to increase blood flow to the brain. Vitamin B-12 helps to promote the function of healthy brain cells and can decrease irritability and depression. L-Tryptophan is a precursor of the essential brain chemical, serotonin, which helps to induce sleep and promotes a positive mood. In a clinical study of 38 healthy women, tryptophan was shown to have "increased the recognition of happy facial expressions and reduced attentional vigilance towards negative words, and decreased baseline startle responsivity" (Murphy SE et al., Psychopharmacology (Berl, 2006), and the depletion of tryptophan and phenylalanine (also in HAPPYTM) in healthy women "increases vulnerability to lowered mood" (Leveton, 2000). Glycine helps reduce anxiety and can give the blissful feeling that some report having after taking alcohol. L-Glutamine is an amino acid found within the actual code of DNA. It is useful to help the body increase its endurance and promote muscle growth.

DREAMS™ was inspired by the drive to promote quality, restful sleep, and pleasant dreams in everyone. **DREAMS** can also be taken to prevent jet lag when used at the beginning of a long flight. Vitamin B-12 helps to maintain healthy nerves and red blood cells and may protect against brain shrinkage while promoting balanced immune functions. Magnesium is used to calm the nervous system. Melatonin is known to have a detoxifying effect, with the right quantities being widely recognized as helping to promote sleep. In a large meta-analysis, melatonin was determined to be "...remarkably effective in preventing or reducing jet-lag" (Herxeimer and Petrie, 2002). Melatonin has been associated with "...increased Actual Sleep Time, Sleep Efficiency, non-REM Sleep, and REM Sleep Latency" (Attenburrow et al. 1996), and has its best effect, comparable to a benzodiazepine sleep aid, when taken between 18.00 - 24.00 h, but not later, because then there is increased secretion of endogenous melatonin (Stone et al., 2000).

IGNITETMwas blended to extend libido and sexual excitement while enhancing performance with its mixed berry taste. Scientifically formulated to increase stamina, blood flow, and staying power, it features ingredients like vitamin E, an important antioxidant; and chromium, which is an essential trace element that can help manage blood sugar as part of a healthy diet and helps promote a healthy libido. Ginseng Root Extract promotes nitric oxide to help sustain sexual function. Oat Straw Extract promotes energy and excitement. Epimedium Grass Extract has reported aphrodisiac effects. N-Acetyl-L-Tyrosine increases drive and enhances energy. Yohimbine Hydrochloride enhances vasodilation in men and engorgement in women. L-Arginine is an amino acid that supports healthy recovery, which, when combined with other herbals, was demonstrated, in a clinical study, to "significantly improve sexual function" (Bottari et al., 2013). When combined with yohimbine, it was associated with "substantially increased vaginal pulse amplitude responses to an erotic film at 60 minutes post-drug administration compared with placebo" (Meston and Worcel, 2002), and improving erectile function in men with mild dysfunction (Akhondzadeh et al., 2010).

Astronuff was the first to speak this time, whilst stroking his shaggy beard, after a sizeable period of reflection. He remembered working with John at Oxford on some of the ideas related to dietary precursors like tryptophan, and also, complex experiments to examine the effects of selective dietary nutrients on brain function. Astronuff knew that most brain chemicals needed to be in the right state and balance for optimal function, and that the depletion of certain nutrients, using the brain-barrier concept, could result in powerful effects on mood. Indeed, it has been demonstrated that if you provide a meal with large amino acids but deficient in tryptophan, which is the precursor for the mood stabilizer, serotonin, found in the brain, then these amino acids are taken up preferentially. If done early in the morning, individuals vulnerable to low moods are gloomy by mid-morning and literally bawling their eyes out by early afternoon, if not sooner. All of this could be corrected rapidly by a large dose of l-tryptophan

Astronuff also knew that l-tryptophan levels are associated with the stabilization of not only mood but also cognition, and that new theories were emerging on gut-brain axis mechanisms to elevate moods and general well-being.

"Well, you have been busy in your spare time," stated Astronuff. "I will not debate the merits of giving supplements to people with deficiencies because that is obvious. Vitamins are essential to maintain good health, and because the body does not make most of them, they have to be ingested. The real question is whether these supplements help individuals who are healthy, and for how long?"

John was expecting this question, but before he could answer, Pamela jumped in.

"Some say all this vitamin-taking is just a placebo, and actually started in earnest with Dr. John Myers in Baltimore. There are very few studies on vitamins supercharging you, even though many celebrities seem to swear by it, especially the rapid infusions".

John put down his teacup and loosened his collar. These were important questions from really smart people that he respected.

The answer came readily. "I applaud that you are looking at this question in terms of a null hypothesis, which, stated simply, means you start with assuming there is no difference between two conditions, and you have to prove that your active condition is better than the placebo condition. But there are many assumptions in those statements that we truly do forget. For instance, we assume the people in any comparative conditions are similar on the basis of simply measured parametric biological variables like age, weight, gender, and the like; however, can we truly balance their expectancies?"

Receiving no reply, he continued. "Experiments are also done with a certain set of quantified variables - like, you are expected to turn up on a certain day at a particular time - whilst the experiment of life is ongoing. It's quasi-experimental. Those parameters of expectancy are not re-balanced every time a person turns up for an experiment, but the expectation is that there is a randomness to this effect, and if a large number of people are sampled, the randomness will be evenly distributed between the groups. That is, in and of itself, a powerful assumption."

Pushing back in his chair until he almost fell out of it, Astronuff became quite provocative, having no intention to fall behind or lose the argument.

"John, is this some kind of casuistry based argument?" he barked.

John maintained his composure and responded more politely than Astronuff deserved.

"I am not a lawyer, nor am I a disciple of Aristotle(384-322 BC) who was famous for casuistry-based arguments. But as you know, the term casuistry has been most abused by those who do not fully understand it. You should read the book by Albert Jonsen and Stephen Toulmin on the abuse of casuistry,26 if you have not already".

"Steady on, boys. This is just us chatting science. No need to get into philosophy, or worse, religion, which are not our specialties. Can we get back to the science? And John, what are your thoughts on Astronuff's posits?" Pamela said wisely, but the upturned corner of her lip and the glint in her eye revealed she was really up to mischief. She had cast down the gauntlet between Astronuff and John, and appointed herself the referee in one fell swoop; like high noon in a spaghetti western. Pamela had perched herself in a no-risk position, where she could preside and rule.

How smart of her, John reflected later on, *to be the 'good', whilst Astronuff and I fought over who was the 'bad', and who the 'ugly'.*

Presently, John thought momentarily before he responded.

"An important part of the supposition is his word 'healthy'. Many of us really aren't particularly healthy, and most of us do not have anything close to a wholesome diet. Vitamin deficiencies are really very common. Please, allow me to provide some data. Across the pond where I live (i.e., the USA), about 42% of the population is deficient in vitamin D. Eighty to 90% of vegetarians and vegans are deficient in vitamin B12.[27] Therefore, that healthy person in your description is less common than you think, and I have not even mentioned how common deficiencies in trace minerals like selenium, chromium, and magnesium really are! How often do these "healthy" people run a panel for full vitamin levels unless they are not feeling their best? Very few, I would propose."

Astronuff replied, "I will give you that, John, but is this also region-specific?"

"Funny you should ask that," John commented, smiling. "If you were to couple the findings on significant amounts of individuals with a vitamin deficiency of one sort or another, and the presence of high-stress - which can be natural like pregnancy or situation-based such as work, school, over-indulging in alcohol or other substances, partying often, and basically burning the candle at both ends - you would see that a significant portion of the population is vulnerable. Additionally, the smart use of supplements to treat "symptoms", if done sensibly, can be an important part of holistic treatment plans for many. Finally, an easy way to give vitamins can be intravenously, but you have to be careful not to administer a significant overdose as that too may cause health problems."

Pamela interrupted.

"Alright then, this is what I understand so far: We are not advocating to give vitamin supplements to completely healthy people who are not in a high demand situation or pressurized setting and whose level of immunity is normal. Nor for those who not overindulge in any way, be it alcohol, drugs, substances, or partying. We do not seek to give these supplements to people who eat a perfectly balanced omnivore diet, have no significant health problems that can affect or alter vitamin levels, or those who regularly check their vitamin levels."

John and Astronuff nodded in agreement.

"Rather," she expounded, "what we are contesting is what constitutes 'healthy' and the approach to it. Astronuff is advocating that healthy to him means the absence of serious disease, while John uses the term to define an "optimum state" of physical health and emotional balance. John is also saying that by his definition, there is a significant portion of people who could not be defined as healthy in the western world and that these people might benefit from supplements. This benefit only applies where it can be done in proper doses. The route of administration, be it oral, intravenous, or a combination of the two, is a choice between the physician and the client." She looked around again, and meeting no dissent, continued.

"Finally, John pointed out that expectancy is important. For many, the word 'expectancy' or 'placebo' is almost like a dirty word. Something ineffective, and a waste of time. But in reality, expectancy is a very powerful tool in medicine; some say it is the best drug ever invented. All doctors rely on the fact that the people who come to see them want to be "better", to aid the process of their recovery. Indeed, the opposite is not typically observed (except in the case of some mental illnesses), whereby the client goes to see their doctor with the expectation of promoting a deterioration in their condition. Thus, this area of supplementation is a difficult one to study empirically."

Pamela rose from her chair, which prompted John and Astronuff to do the same.

"Follow me boys! Time for a beer and an unhealthy bacon sandwich for lunch!" she commanded and disappeared outside into the blazing sun.

Signature Note: The Body Adapts - So Can You

John, reflecting on his walk past Magdalen College years later, remembered how the 2019 Nobel Prize in Physiology or Medicine honored William G. Kaelin Jr., Sir Peter J. Ratcliffe, and Gregg L. Semenza for revealing how cells sense and adapt to oxygen availability—a reminder that survival is often decided in quiet, molecular choices long before it is visible on the surface.

Chapter 6

Some Concluding Remarks To Book 1 of 3

You've reached the close of Book 1 - where restoration begins, and where the idea of brain wellness becomes personal.

Through John's experiences, you've seen how early wounds can echo into adulthood - and how insight, support, and deliberate practice can soften their grip.

You've also explored a central question: what does it mean to keep a brain not only "healthy," but truly well - steady in mood, clear in thinking, and resilient under stress?

Finally, you've been introduced to a foundational principle of recovery: for many people struggling with alcohol or drugs, nutritional and medical support is not optional - it is part of giving the brain a fair chance to heal.

In Book 2, the lens widens. You'll step into evaluative personalization - where treatment becomes tailored, evidence becomes actionable, and your story matters as much as your symptoms.

Chapter 7

Further Reading and References

Johnson BA, Roache JD, eds. *Drug addiction and its treatment: nexus of neuroscience and behavior*. Philadelphia, PA: Lippincott-Raven Publishers; 1997.

Johnson BA, Ruiz P, Galanter M, eds. *Handbook of clinical alcoholism treatment*. Baltimore: Lippincott Williams & Wilkins; 2003.

Johnson BA, ed. *Addiction medicine: science and practice*. New York: Springer Science+Business Media; 2010.

Johnson BA, Roache JD, Javors MA, DiClemente CC, Cloninger CR, Prihoda TJ, Bordnick PS, Ait-Daoud N, Hensler J. Ondansetron for reduction of drinking among biologically predisposed alcoholic patients: a randomized controlled trial. *JAMA*. 2000;284:963-971.

Johnson BA, Ait-Daoud N, Bowden CL, DiClemente CC, Roache JD, Lawson K, Javors MA, Ma JZ. Oral topiramate for treatment of alcohol dependence: a randomized controlled trial. *Lancet*. 2003;361:1677-1685.

Johnson BA, Rosenthal N, Capece JA, Wiegand F, Mao L, Beyers K, McKay A, Ait-Daoud N, Anton RF, Ciraulo DA, Kranzler HR, Mann K, O'Malley SS, Swift RM, Topiramate for Alcoholism Advisory Board, Topiramate for Alcoholism Study Group. Topiramate for treating alcohol dependence: a randomized controlled trial. *JAMA*. 2007;298:1641-1651.

Anton RF, O'Malley SS, Ciraulo DA, Cisler RA, Couper D, Donovan DM, Gastfriend DR, Hosking JD, Johnson BA, LoCastro JS, Longabaugh R, Mason BJ, Mattson ME, Miller WR, Pettinati HM, Randall CL, Swift R, Weiss RD, Williams LD, Zweben A, COMBINE Study Research Group. Combined pharmacotherapies and behavioral interventions for alcohol dependence - The COMBINE Study: a randomized controlled trial. *JAMA*. 2006;295:2003-2017.

Johnson BA, Ait-Daoud N, Seneviratne C, Roache JD, Javors MA, Wang X-Q, Liu L, Penberthy JK, DiClemente CC, Li MD. Pharmacogenetic approach at the serotonin transporter gene as a method of reducing the severity of alcohol drinking. *Am J Psychiatry*. 2011;168:265-275.

Johnson, BA. Addiction Medicine. Published by Elsevier, 2019

Chapter 8

BOOK 2: Evaluative Personalization

Now we move from principles to interventions—from insight to treatment.

This second book in the *Six Rings* series focuses on **"Evaluative Personalization"**—a framework for matching addiction treatments to the individual, using evidence-based assessment and (at its most advanced) **pharmacogenetics** (genetics-informed medication selection). It's written as **story-driven clinical parables** that weave in neuroscience, practical treatment principles, and "myth-busting" about addiction and recovery.

Chapter 9

Introduction
To Book 2 of 3

Evaluative personalization is a term coined by Professor Dr. Bankole A. Johnson to describe a simple but radical idea: treatment should be built around the person - not forced upon them.

At its core, personalization means gathering the many factors that shape a person's experience - biology, history, environment, habits, trauma, strengths - and letting that full picture guide care.

In modern addiction medicine, one promising frontier is pharmacogenetics: using a person's genetic profile to match them with the medication most likely to help.

In practice, this can look as straightforward as a blood test followed by a tailored prescription - yet the science beneath it is extraordinary, and still evolving.

Within Six Rings, The Professor extends this idea through Deep Behavioral Phenotyping (DBP): a structured way to understand patterns of behavior with greater depth and humility.

Because human beings are complex, the work is complex. But complexity is not the enemy - confusion is. This book aims to make advanced concepts feel usable.

The stories that follow introduce big ideas in approachable ways, so you can absorb the science without losing the human thread.

Unlike Book 1, John is not always at the center—and that is intentional. Some lessons are best learned by watching from the edge. When John does appear, he carries both the rigor of a physician-scientist and the method of a forensic examiner, learning to reconstruct cause, sequence, and motive without losing compassion.

Each major section opens with a brief evidence-based discussion of a substance use disorder, followed by stories that make the data personal - and the personal actionable.

If you've been reading along, you are already learning more than facts. You are learning a way of thinking - curious, compassionate, and precise.

Alcohol Use Disorder:

Some Myths, Some Answers

What Do We Know Now?

For many, the disease of alcohol use disorder follows a chronic relapsing course. We do, however, know that for many, it is an episodic disease during which "attacks" can be interspersed with long periods, sometimes even years, of remission, or *vice versa*. However, not all those with alcohol use disorder follow the same path. For some, it is like having diabetes, with the disease being present all the time, but displaying periodic exacerbations. For others, it is more like asthma, which can be severe at times of an "attack," but an individual can be free of its prominent symptoms for lengthy periods. And more still, it is like having High Blood Pressure - present most of the time, but "controllable" with the right treatment. Whether it is psychological, social, or genealogical factors that influence a person to embrace alcoholism doesn't really matter; the primary disorder that provokes excessive drinking is in the brain, and it is that organ that is the target for treatments to curb the disease.

Nevertheless, excessive drinking and alcohol use disorder can be accompanied by serious health problems in other organs. These include gastrointestinal disorders with ulcers and bleeding; liver disease and its eventual failure; a poorly functioning heart and related diseases including High Blood Pressure, increased cholesterol, and heart attacks; many cancers; vitamin deficiencies and brittle bones that can lead to fractures. In the brain, there could be dementia, confusion, visual disturbance, hallucinations (hearing voices or seeing things that are not there), and delusions (false beliefs that, when of a paranoid nature, increase the risk of violence to the person and others). Indeed, alcohol use disorder can be associated with over one hundred serious medical illnesses.

A recent World Health Organization report ranks the disorder as the leading cause of morbidity and mortality for individuals between 15 to 49 years - meant to be their most productive years - in the world. Binge drinking increases the above-enumerated risks and goes mostly untreated because of poor screening, primarily in general health care clinics and centers.

The propensity to drink excessively and to develop a problem with alcohol is controlled by several genes, the exact nature of which has not been fully revealed. Nevertheless, we do know that the genetic contribution toward developing alcoholism is about 60%, with psychosocial determinants making up the other 40%. It is important to know that the rates of genetic risk for developing asthma, diabetes, and high blood pressure are similar and are all diseases that are well established as medical issues. So, it seems strange that a common myth about alcohol use disorder is that it is not a medical disease. Those individuals might argue that the individual who develops alcohol use disorder can "control" it by simply refusing to drink. That is, however, a false argument as many human diseases with a genetic component also has an aspect that can be "controlled", yet individuals with those diseases are not blamed for developing them.

A Case in point is those with genetic risks for asthma, diabetes, and High Blood Pressure. They can control risk factors such as obesity and smoking with changes in behavior to promote health. That does not, however, mean that should they not succeed entirely, or if they end up developing the disease anyway, that their illness will be tagged not medical in nature. Obviously, it would be wise to counsel people with family histories of alcoholism (and at high risk genetically) to reduce their risk by choosing to limit their exposure to alcohol use. Gainsaying this, that can be easier said than done. The advice, whilst sensible at face value, may be hard to achieve because people with a biological propensity towards the disease are "driven" to use it not only by their genes but also by environmental factors.

The way The Professor illustrates it to his students is thus:

Let's say your plane crashed in a desert, and you were the only survivor. You are thirsty and stumble upon an oasis but notice from the carcasses of dead animals around the body of water that it must be poisoned. At first, perhaps a full day, your rational self will not attempt to drink from it. Eventually however, as your thirst becomes intolerable, you will eventually attempt to drink from the pool - perhaps hoping that your initial conclusion that it was poisoned might not entirely be true, or simply feeling compelled to drink the water. It matters not the over-riding reason, the point to be noted here is that this same cycle of compulsion and choices is often faced by individuals with alcohol use disorder. So, whilst your genes are not your destiny, when combined with an adverse environment that conditions behavior, the compulsion is hard to resist, and it'd seem like there are no good options to avoid the inevitable outcome.

It is difficult for many young people to make responsible decisions about their health. Some aren't capable of deciding between right and wrong on such simple tasks as eating, sleeping, studying, or driving. The reason is both biological and environmental. Science teaches that the executive functions of the brain (i.e., those that are involved with thinking and judging consequences) are not developed fully until the early '20s, and most individuals younger than that age do not have sufficient experience with the power of consequences to shape behavior. When they attempt to understand their world, a good number of young people see a society that encourages individuals to use alcohol as a means to feel good. Once they start to drink heavily, what happens down the line is largely influenced by an individual's genetic vulnerability to alcohol abuse and the way that person's body and mind react to alcohol.

On the simplest level, men and women process alcohol differently. The bodies of women generally don't tolerate alcohol as well as men's do. Women tend to weigh less, have a smaller volume of blood, and have a lower ratio of body water to body fat, meaning their bodies do not break alcohol down as efficiently. These disparities often lead women to develop alcohol-related medical problems more quickly than men. Strangely enough, because of the stigma associated with seeking treatment, women tend to arrive later into treatment than men and can present a more severe alcohol use disorder pattern.

Ethnicity can help spare some people from developing alcoholism. Up to 35 percent of Chinese and Japanese people have a genetic variation in the gene that breaks down alcohol (i.e., alcohol dehydrogenase), which causes unpleasant sensations and makes their skin flush when they drink alcohol. People who experience such physical reactions tend to be discouraged from drinking. Research is ongoing, and remains unclear, as to whether certain genetic predispositions that provoke excessive drinking may be more common in different ethnic populations.

Sons of alcoholic fathers often have a higher tolerance for alcohol than the general population. Many can drink more without getting drunk or experiencing a hangover. That increased capacity for alcohol means that this group has to consume more alcohol to experience its pleasurable effects.

Therefore, brain chemistry among this group actually promotes heavier drinking.

Animal studies have shown that alcohol changes the brain's "reward" circuitry by stimulating the dopamine system (the so-called "pleasure center" of the brain) and other associated brain regions, which leads to intense compulsive behaviors that can make lab rats pass over their basic needs for food and water in their quest to drink more alcohol. Important to note is that not all compulsive behaviors are "pleasurable", and in humans who are addicted to alcohol or drugs, the compulsion is not, typically, described as pleasurable but more motoric in quality.

But the brain doesn't return to normal after a person with alcohol use disorder stops drinking. Even if they've stopped drinking long enough to end a physical dependence on alcohol, they will usually continue to crave it. This is because the memory of their craving is stored in the brain and can be re-activated fully with renewed excessive drinking. Many, but not all, with alcohol use disorder crave alcohol even though they realize drinking will mess up their lives. This phenomenon, romantically coined the *"dark side"* of addiction, may explain why so many people relapse after achieving abstinence, and the targeting of this biological abnormality using effective medicines is a new approach being developed to curb alcohol use disorder.

People who drink heavily over long periods may suffer short and long-term brain damage. Heavy drinking also may affect a person's 'survival' circuitry, that part of the brain responsible for motivation, appetite, emotions, and memory. Survival circuitry provides the instinct to avoid danger. Heavy drinking over time can alter brain chemistry and leave behind psychological conditioning that limits a person's ability to control the desire to drink.

So, for some people with alcohol use disorder, the act of drinking becomes wired into the survival circuitry. It literally takes control of the brain. Just the smell of beer, the recollection of a favorite bar, or any other cue can make an alcoholic crave drinking as strongly as hunger and thirst make everyone else crave food and water.

Some people with alcohol use disorder do not crave alcohol in the typical sense. These individuals seem to drink in a more driven and motoric manner in order to avoid "negative emotions" when they are drinking (typically of anxiety or depression), or at times, just to remedy the state of "not feeling alive". These individuals who use alcohol excessively to avoid negative emotions tend to have more co-morbid psychiatric disorders and require more complex treatments.

So How Does an individual with Alcohol Use Disorder Get Better?

For years, the prevailing theory about how individuals with alcohol use disorder could overcome the craving for alcohol was simple: All they had to do was *talk* about it. A lot. Every day. Often, with others who also had issues with alcohol abuse. Sometimes, they had to confess their sins, repent for past misdeeds, make reparations, and seek divine guidance. Though some benefited from these self-help methods, using this approach to the exclusion of treating the underlying disease is like fighting with one hand tied behind your back.

There are many anecdotes in alcohol recovery. Phrases like

'one day at a time' are often used to focus on trying to maintain sobriety in incremental time units. If a person feels the urge to drink, they should "neither yield nor resist", but merely put off that particular drink until the next day. This delay in segregating the thoughts about alcohol and the consequences of drinking is supposed to help fade the memory of drinking. The problem with this is that we know that the brain stores these memories, perhaps interminably, and thus not drinking is merely inhibiting the behavioral expression of the disease.

Without adding medication to psychosocial treatment, 70 percent of individuals may resume drinking within one year. But then, psychosocial intervention alone - be it full-blown psychotherapy or the lifelong "commitment" required by self-help groups - is not an optimal treatment for alcohol use disorder. Remember, 60 percent of the alcohol use disorder is driven by biology. Thus, simply working on the remaining 40 percent that is environmentally determined is, inarguably, an incomplete treatment.

On any given day, more than a quarter of a million Americans who seek help for an alcohol problem can't get it. They seek help through rehab centers or detoxification programs or other means, but as it happens, they either can't afford them, don't have the insurance coverage, or simply don't know where to go. And up to 90 percent of people with serious drinking problems never get formal treatment at all.

The more we know about treating alcohol use disorder, the more we know that those failure statistics should shrink exponentially. The need for intensive psychotherapy or formally structured long-term alcohol counseling is becoming a thing of the past. Many studies demonstrate that intensive psychotherapy is even less effective than brief intervention plus a placebo pill. For alcohol treatment, there is little evidence to show that simply intensifying psychological treatment is related directly to more favorable outcomes. Targeted psychosocial support with medicines or other active interventions seems more likely to succeed.

Research shows that brief interventions, such as Brief Behavioral Compliance Enhancement Treatment (BBCET), Medical Management (MM), and a model called BRENDA, have been shown to optimize the treatment of alcohol use disorder when used with effective medications. Brief motivational treatments have also been found to be helpful.

There is no longer a clinical rationale to delay providing medications to help individuals with alcohol use disorder. Additionally, personalizing the medical approach is most likely to result in the best outcomes. Some medical professionals still believe in the theory that they should not dispense medication until lengthy sessions of psychotherapy or self-help have begun. Now, a brief psychosocial and effective intervention can be provided by physicians in general practice.

Blowing Away Traditional Myths

The expectation that an individual with alcohol use disorder must be completely sober before treatment can begin has dominated treatment philosophies for about 100 years. This goes along with a popular perception usually associated with treating just about any addiction, that a person has to hit "rock bottom" before they can bounce back.

In fact, when people are faced with nothing more to lose, they may find themselves hurtling further toward "the bottom." One study concluded that involuntary job loss is linked to subsequent increases in alcohol consumption among those who had been non-drinkers. Conversely, people in the study who had a history of alcohol consumption experienced no substantial change in alcohol intake after losing their jobs. Also, it was concluded that people who began drinking after an involuntary job loss did so twice as often as employed people.

The conclusion of this study may reinforce a long-held perception that people of higher incomes fare better in treatment because they have more to lose. But it may also simply be that people in higher income brackets can come up with the high fees charged by private rehabilitation centers. They may be able to continue coming up with those fees over and over since the medium-term failure rate for people who attend such institutions is very high.

So, do you need to hit rock bottom, lose your job, family, house, and whatever little self-esteem you have remaining before you can *begin* to get better?

You might be able to recover on your own.

There is an appreciating percentage of individuals with alcohol use disorder who recover on their own, without drugs or behavioral treatment. Some people who had been heavy drinkers in college find that the demands of work and family leave them with little time or inclination to drink much anymore. Studies show that drinking problems and the amount of alcohol consumed often decrease in men after the age of 50 years. The overall rate of spontaneous remission has been reported at about 5 percent per year. That means in any one year, 5 percent of all people who have alcohol problems will stop drinking on their own for at least 12 months. But again, do you *have to* wait until things get worse *before* things can get better?

You'd be hard-pressed to find anyone in the U.S. treatment community who would argue that abstinence is not the best possible outcome for an individual with alcohol use disorder. But in other parts of the world, the idea of "harm reduction," which is basically moderation, is far more embraced than it is in the U.S.

Moderation advocates embrace the idea that controlled drinking is actually more likely to help an individual reach sobriety than the *holy grail* of 'all-or-nothing.' Often, an individual with alcohol use disorder will choose 'all' rather than 'nothing'. As many as 80 percent of individuals with alcohol use disorder either can't or won't stop drinking. If these people aren't given the option to drink moderately and reduce the harm, those handling treatments are missing out on opportunities to help them feel differently so that they can progress toward abstinence.

The "Leap" to Science

New discoveries on how to change the way a brain responds to alcohol are being developed rapidly. The change in how we approach the accumulation of neuroscientific knowledge may finally eliminate alcohol use disorder. These new discoveries may help put to rest the notion that *only* lots and lots of talking will help those with alcohol use disorder get better.

As a leader in the development of clinical trials for

topiramate, one of the new classes of drugs that can help people put aside the craving to drink, the Professor found that people could begin taking the drug even while they were still drinking. The same goes for another medicine he discovered - ultra-low-dose ondansetron- which is used to treat individuals with a specific genetic pattern who have alcohol use disorder.

His obstinacy in developing this approach to treating individuals who were, at the time, using alcohol excessively was not without consequences. Pioneers can often have a difficult time. Having endured all sorts of opposition, including the receipt of open death threats, letters to his university employers to dismiss him, a multitude of books from religious agencies seeking to change his views, and disparaging articles, there is now a deep feeling of vindication in him as, over the years, ideas have seen fulfillment.

As a safety catch, practically no new medicinal treatments for alcohol use disorder are tested on people who are still drinking, or who are susceptible to resume their drinking in a "high-risk" situation.

Part of this research was conducted while Prof. Dr. Bankole A. Johnson was in the faculty at the University of Texas. At that school's San Antonio medical center, he ran a walk-in clinic for individuals with alcohol use disorder. People would simply wander in off the street and begin their evaluation, followed by treatment if they were eligible to participate in the study.

The rate of success we had by giving people topiramate and another medicine, ondansetron, was remarkable! People were literally changing their habits of drinking a couple of bottles of wine a day to drinking about a couple of glasses.

And, these people were making progress without first having to be sent to a specialist or a detoxification clinic at the cost of thousands of dollars (often money that they didn't have anyway). When a doctor can prescribe medicine for an individual with alcohol use disorder during his or her first visit to the office, without the need to dry out first, it means a huge barrier to treatment has been removed.

One of the most amazing success stories told about the Professor's time at the University of Texas studying the effects of topiramate involved a gentleman who'd had alcohol use disorder for a very long time. He'd tried any number of self-help groups and been to rehab several times, but would remark that whenever he had a session, all the talk of alcohol made him "thirsty".

The man's wife finally had enough and confronted him with a demand that he gets treatment. In trying to avoid her wrath, he had actually contemplated jumping out of a window. The injuries he could have sustained might have killed him.

Once he was enrolled in our study, he improved, stopped drinking, and basically became the "poster child" for topiramate. By the time the Professor left the University of Texas for a position at the University of Virginia, the man had been sober for five years - the longest time he hadn't had a drink in his adult life.

Alcohol use disorder may never be curable with just a pill; behavioral elements and medical conditions that contribute to the disease, such as depression, often need to be figured out simultaneously. But without acknowledging the significant role that medications can have in helping the brain of an individual with alcohol use disorder overcome its faulty circuitry, the opportunity to help a majority of the people in the world with the disease might not occur.

The COMBINE Study

One of the most significant clinical trials to demonstrate the effectiveness of medications that help people recover from alcoholism is the Combining Medications and Behavioral Interventions for Alcoholism (COMBINE) study. It represents the largest clinical trial ever done by the United States National Institutes of Health (NIH) on pharmacological and behavioral treatments for alcohol use disorder.

The results of this NIH run study were released in 2006. Results showed that the medication naltrexone, when accompanied with brief counseling, was the most effective method for curtailing drinking and enhancing abstinence among alcoholics. It also proved that if a "slip" did occur, a person would ultimately still drink less. What was fascinating about this study was that the individuals who received no pills, but just a highly intensive psychotherapy program called Combined Behavioral Intervention, had the worst clinical outcomes, were most likely to relapse, and stuck with treatment the least. A lot of talking, no matter how targeted and even when delivered by experts, was no better than a placebo pill with brief counseling.

Furthermore, with as many as 90 percent of people who have alcohol use disorder not getting any treatment, the study showed that even those with severe alcohol problems could be treated on an outpatient basis. Essentially, this study added to the growing evidence that the treatment for drinking disorders could be implemented in a variety of health care settings, including the offices of family physicians and mental health care providers. The availability of medicines to deal with alcohol use disorder dramatically expands access to effective treatment, and it offers individuals greater treatment choices.

Not All Heavy Drinkers Are the Same

Alcoholics may potentially fall into at least two different subtypes; early-onset and late-onset alcoholism. Some experts, however, believe that there could be other subtypes both within and distinct from each category, as well as other types that can be defined more specifically with the advancement of molecular genetics techniques.

Early-onset alcohol use disorder is characterized by a strong family history of alcohol use disorder, a broad range of impulse-control problems and traits, and early onset (before the age of 25) of problem drinking. Late-onset alcohol use disorder is characterized by a later age at the onset of problem drinking (typically at age 25 or older) and a higher rate of psychosocial problems, combined with little or no family history of alcoholism. When a doctor assesses the degree of alcohol use disorder, figuring out the individual's subtype may depend on knowing at what age the individual recognized that drinking was a problem. It seems that different types of medication (such as a class of drugs often associated with depression known as Selective Serotonin Reuptake Inhibitors - SSRIs) that act on a brain chemical called serotonin may be effective in treating a particular subtype of alcohol use disorder.

More encouraging still is the knowledge that research on

medications that affect the serotonin system is becoming more exciting. The potential to identify genetic markers that may help to determine who should get specific types of medication is now present. That potential also includes being able to monitor changes in proteins made by these genetic markers to see the progress a medicine is making. Imagine having a problem with alcohol, going to your doctor for help, getting a genetic test, and then being prescribed a medication that is just right for you. Such an example is described in a paper that was published in *The American Journal of Psychiatry* in March 2011, entitled "Pharmacogenetic Approach at the Serotonin Transporter Gene as a Method of Reducing the Severity of Alcohol Drinking". [overview] That is the future of treatment through medication for alcoholism, and it heralds the arrival of personalized or precision medicine.

Often concurrent with alcohol use is the condition of depression. This was proven in an NIAAA study called the National Epidemiologic Survey on Alcohol and Related Conditions (NESARC), which followed 43,000 adults. The rate of alcohol use disorders was 14 percent amongst participants with a 12-month history of major depressive disorder. The incidence of alcohol use disorders among people with a lifetime history of depression was 40 percent.

The NESARC findings suggest a genetic link between a propensity for alcohol use disorder and depression. For instance, older women who live alone may be particularly prone to alcohol misuse and depression resulting from loneliness. Symptoms of depression frequently arise among people who have alcohol dependence (especially during withdrawal when problems with insomnia, anxiety, and mood dips can complicate recovery). What the NESARC results mean is that all doctors who treat individuals with alcohol use disorder should examine them for symptoms of depression.

Another disturbing trend has been the increase in hazardous drinking among adolescents and young adults. Often referred to as binge drinking, the incidence remains frequent among those of college age, despite increased prevention efforts.

The problem with identifying binge drinkers is that physicians tend to be less thorough in asking questions that might uncover those tendencies. A younger patient may present with excellent physical health, and, therefore, a doctor may not even ask about alcohol consumption or screen the patient for alcohol problems. But among the top 10 high-risk drinking populations in the U.S., about half are young adults. Asking questions, giving advice, or leading a brief formal intervention may save lives in the short term and reduce risks of health problems that develop later, such as alcohol-related organ damage.

A survey called the Behavior Risk Factor Surveillance System (BRFSS), which is analyzed by the Centers for Disease Control and Prevention (CDC), is a collection of data on health risk behaviors, clinical preventive practices, and health care access as related to chronic diseases and injury. The BRFSS reveals some disturbing trends in alcohol use among people aged 18 and older.

About 44 percent of students attending four-year colleges say they drink in binges, according to a 2005 topic review published in the *Southern Medical Journal* called *Alcohol on*

Trial: The Evidence. College students are more likely to become binge drinkers when exposed to places where alcohol is accessible, abundant, and cheap. Between 1993 and 2001, binge-drinking episodes in the U.S. increased from 1.2 billion to 1.5 billion. Binge drinking episodes per person per year also grew 17.3 percent over the same time frame. Men account for 81 percent of binge-drinking episodes. This form of alcohol consumption is common among young adults, but 69 percent of all individual binge drinking episodes occur in people older than age 25.

On the positive side, brief intervention programs have proven successful in reducing alcohol intake among heavy-drinking college students. Information on these students, as well as the effectiveness of specific interventions, was presented at a 2003 meeting of the Research Society on Alcoholism and was recounted in a 2004 edition of *Alcoholism: Clinical & Experimental Research*. Various brief interventions were described by the authors, including; group classroom sessions, individual Motivational Intervention (MI), and one-on-one or computerized alcohol education.

The students who entered a brief intervention program when they were still drinking frequently and heavily experienced reductions in their long-term alcohol consumption and fewer negative consequences as a result of their drinking. Those who received MI had counseling on alcohol-related problems, situations associated with heavy drinking, personal consumption, and drinking levels that they perceived as being normal. At follow-up visits, they reported reductions in weekly alcohol consumption, binge drinking, and overall drinking frequency.

MI is a collaborative, non-confrontational way of addressing drinking behavior. It can be effective with emerging adults, especially those who are more likely to resist confrontations that seem authoritarian. MI assesses the motivation that a student has to curtail drinking, and then tailors the intervention accordingly. If a student is drinking heavily, has had many negative consequences as a result, but still seems to give little thought to changing this behavior, MI focuses on increasing awareness of these negative consequences along with their current and future risks.

Being cost-effective and led by trained non-professionals (at times, even other undergraduate college students), this method may increase the odds that those being counseled will seek additional help. MI can be partnered with something called "booster sessions". This is the time the student being counseled can raise issues not addressed in the first MI session, or revisit topics that warrant more discussion. Booster sessions also provide opportunities to discuss alcohol-related experiences that have occurred in the interim.

Most importantly, among the populations examined, brief interventions such as MI succeeded where most other interventional approaches that had been used and studied failed. Continued research is looking at ways to add effective medicines to MI to enhance the chances of treating adolescents and emerging adults successfully.

Some Science about the Alcohol Use Disordered Brain

Advances in neuroscience are helping researchers to study how and when the repeated chemical interaction of alcohol with the brain causes addiction in some people but not others. This research will eventually aid the understanding of why some people can't control their drinking after a certain point, and why these people require increasing quantities of alcohol to feel its euphoric effects.

The central factor by which people experience the effects of alcohol is principally dopamine, a chemical in the brain that is a neurotransmitter. Neurotransmitters are chemicals manufactured by the brain that relay, amplify, and modulate signals between nerve cells (neurons) and other cells. Dopamine affects brain processes that control movement, emotions, and the ability to experience pleasure and pain. The way dopamine is regulated in the brain can help determine a person's mental and physical health.

Neurons that contain dopamine run from a region in the back of the brain (called the ventral tegmental area), to a relay center at about the middle (called the nucleus accumbens), and then to the front parts of the brain (the orbitofrontal cortex). These neurons play a big part in how the rewarding effects of alcohol are expressed. This circuit is also termed the cortico-mesolimbic dopamine system. In this "reward" circuit, the drive to consume alcohol is integrated with memories and emotions about a person's prior alcohol use (particularly in certain settings) and feeds this information to the cortex. The cortex then makes a 'go/no-go' decision whether or not more alcohol should be consumed. What we are finding out is that this reward circuit does not function independently, but is fine-tuned by many other neurotransmitter systems. Notable among these systems that modulate the reward circuit are those which contain gamma-aminobutyric acid (GABA), glutamate (GLU), serotonin (5-HT), opioids, and smaller molecules such as neurokinins.

The following explains the roles and functions of GABA, glutamate, serotonin, neurokinins, and other small molecules:

GABA

GABA is the leading inhibitory neurotransmitter in the central nervous system (CNS). It plays a role in regulating a neuron's ability to receive and respond to a stimulus throughout the CNS. Alcohol modulates the effect of GABA receptors and increases the inhibitory or "quieting" effect that GABA has on neurons. GABA receptors are in many parts of the brain, and GABA accounts for alcohol's sedating effect on many brain functions, including judgment, movement, and breathing.

Prolonged alcohol use may cause the brain to adapt and become dependent on the presence of alcohol to function normally. When a heavy drinker stops drinking, the lack of alcohol attached to GABA leads to increased anxiety, jitteriness, emotional discomfort, insomnia, and maybe even some tremors. Medicines designed to reduce the withdrawal effects of alcohol typically have effects on the GABA system.

Glutamate

Glutamate is one of the brain's most common neurotransmitters, and its main function is to stimulate brain activity. The glutamate system is a fast-signaling system that is important for information processing. Glutamate is also involved in the process of long-term memory.

Research on this system has grown as scientists attempt to understand various neuropsychiatric disorders. Many antipsychotic medicines work on the dopamine system, but glutamate receptors may turn out to be even better targeted for future drugs to treat alcohol use disorder. This is because medicines that work on the glutamate system might essentially help the individual to "unlearn" how to use alcohol excessively or decrease the intensity of the long-term desire to use more alcohol.

Serotonin

Serotonin, or 5-hydroxytryptamine (5-HT), is a neurotransmitter found in the gastrointestinal tract, in blood platelets, and in the CNS. In the CNS, 5-HT helps to regulate appetite, sleep, memory and learning, and mood. Many antidepressant drugs act by regulating serotonin levels in the brain.

The serotonin system in the brain seems to be a central mediator of complex signals in different neuronal pathways. It can do this by modulating the effects of other neurotransmitter systems, including the cortico-mesolimbic dopamine system. Therefore, medications that work in the 5-HT system have been a source of intense research as potential medications to treat alcohol dependence.

Opioids

An opioid is a chemical that can produce a feeling of euphoria. Opioids bind to opioid receptors, which are found mostly in the CNS and the gastrointestinal tract. Opioid receptors in these organ systems mediate between the good effects and (potentially harmful) side effects of opioids. Alcohol use triggers the release of opioids that can lead to the "good effect" of euphoria, but also can be associated with the drowsiness that can ensue from excessive drinking.

The opioid system also affects the cortico-mesolimbic system by fine-tuning its activity and may be associated with hormonal systems that are linked to stress systems that can trigger drinking. Opioid antagonists, such as the drug naltrexone, have been shown to be an effective treatment for alcohol use disorder.

Neurokinins and Small Molecules

The brain contains a tremendous array of small molecules such as neurokinins that can regulate the response to stress, along with hormones to trigger stress-induced excessive alcohol consumption. These stress responses can occur long after the individual with alcohol use disorder has stopped drinking, and then trigger the relapse to resume excessive alcohol consumption. This "dark side" of addiction and how to quell its effects with medicines is a growing area of new research in medicines for treating alcohol use disorder.

*"...beyond science...beyond borders **TM**"*

Evaluative Personalization: Medicines For Addiction

The Answer Man

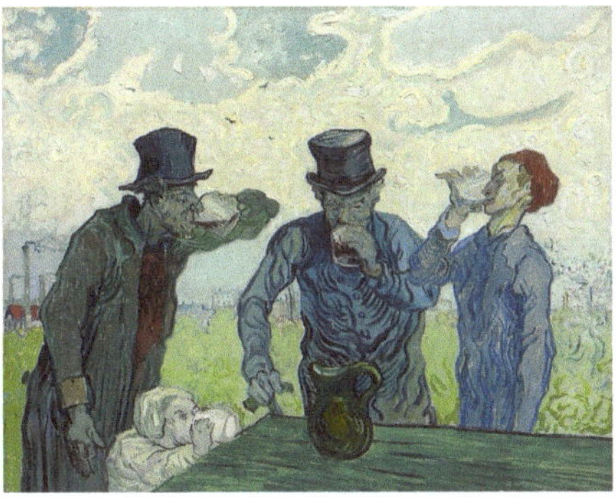

The image above is: The Drinkers - Vincent van Gogh.

Vincent van Gogh's *The Drinkers* borrows its four-stage descent from an earlier Daumier engraving: youth to middle age to collapse. It is an unnerving companion to Pete's arc - a man once called the Answer Man, slowly demoted by alcohol until he is simply the old man in the corner.

Van Gogh floods the scene with sickly greens and blues -

color as chemistry, a hint of absinthe and the way intoxication can turn ordinary hours hallucinatory. Keep that palette in mind: Pete's story shifts from warm competence to a cold, fluorescent haze. (Image courtesy/public domain via the Art Institute of Chicago.)

Pete's story is not about willpower failing. It is about a reward system learning a shortcut. The clinical task is to interrupt the loop - sometimes with psychotherapy, sometimes with medication that blunts reinforcement - before the dragon learns to kill.

Alcohol is an efficient anesthetic for the modern stress response: a fast dopamine signal followed by a slower flood of relief. Over time, the brain starts treating relief as survival. The cue isn't just the bar; it's the calendar invite, the hotel lobby, the first glass pushed across a table.

I have learned to distrust success as a protective factor. The people who can still deliver on Monday often drink the hardest on Friday. Functioning buys time - time to hide, time to bargain, time to tell yourself you're fine.

Harrow's Field Note: The High-Functioning Dragon

For twenty years, Pete was the closer at a supply-distribution firm. In the office, he'd earned the nickname *The Answer Man* - the person who could turn hesitation into signatures.

When leadership needed to win a new account, they sent Pete with charts, projections, and two versions of a client's future.

One spreadsheet traced the status quo: a flat line,

sometimes sliding. The other rose in clean, optimistic angles - the promised lift of a partnership.

He had the degree. He had the patter. He had the timing.

Sealing the Deal

For most of his career, Pete sealed business the old way: a handshake, then a drink. Over lunch, he could read a CFO's posture the way other people read a balance sheet.

If someone hesitated, Pete didn't push harder; he prepared better. Before a meeting, he'd ask an assistant about favorite teams, hobbies - any small loyalty that could open a door. A pair of tickets in an envelope could soften the edges of a negotiation.

If sports weren't the language, he learned another - opera, antiques, movies, food. He wasn't buying people; he was proving he noticed them.

Gift baskets were his harmless superpower. Chocolate, cheese, crackers, a bottle of wine - something inside always became "the best thing we've ever tasted." Even when office policies tightened, Pete could still get a basket past the front desk because he knew the rules well enough to work within them.

"It's fine," Pete would say. "Share it with the team - and don't skip the dark-chocolate coffee beans. They're unbelievable!"

People liked Pete. He dressed sharply, kept a crisp appearance, and wore an everyman ease that made executives feel safe.

But to Pete, it seemed that the tone of business was changing.

Handshakes that used to be firm and strong now felt insincere or weak. Now, contracts had to be considered with RFA (Request for Approval) forms. Confidentiality agreements had to be signed. Meetings had to be conducted with purchasing managers, facilities managers, logistics managers, and, in some cases, even janitors.

What happened to the days when he could just walk into the CEO's office, look him in the eye and say, "Here's what I can do for you"?

Instead of agreeing to meet for lunch to talk over turkey, more clients were e-mailing him with inquiries and requests. He had one client whose preferred method of communication was text messaging, and the guy's office was less than a mile down the road! Pete figured he could probably open a window and yell out his answers in the time it would take him to type half a sentence.

In fact, when he received his first text message on his flip-top model cell phone, he didn't know what was happening. The thing went "bong," and all of a sudden, there were some words flashing on the phone's tiny screen. He had to put on his bifocals to see exactly what it said.

Although he felt embarrassed, he went ahead and asked one of the younger guys in the office what this was. The answer didn't make him feel any better: "That's a text message, old man."

It was stuff like 'text messaging' that was beating Pete down. At age 59, his enthusiasm for work felt stale and clichéd. He wasn't the top guy anymore. His sales figures had dropped in the last two years. It seemed like he was moving in slow motion.

The company was hiring recent college graduates at about one-third of his salary. Pete thought, "Three of them for every one of me? Either I'm that good, or I'm that old."

He wondered how long he could hang on like this. Even his clients were downsizing. One day he'd be talking about office cubicle architecture with a CFO that he'd known for 10 years, the next he'd find himself talking to a junior staff accountant who recently earned an undergraduate degree who was in inventory management.

At 59, he was staring at retirement or maybe being shown the door. Everyone was supposed to be done by 65, when they could sail off into the sunset, secure in the wad of cash they'd packed away over a lifetime.

"Yeah, right," Pete thought. His cynical side was getting the best of him.

Home Sweet Home?

If things weren't bad enough at work, things at home certainly weren't much better.

Pete's wife, Carmen, had become quieter and more withdrawn in the past few years. In fact, it was getting harder for him to see her as the bubbly woman he'd met at a wedding almost 36 years ago.

Carmen was a breast cancer survivor who'd been a shining example of determination to her friends and family. She'd taken treatment head-on, even choosing to participate in a clinical trial. Carmen had emerged from breast cancer with her spirits intact and with a new appreciation for Pete, who'd driven her to every appointment.

For the first six years following her last treatment, Carmen seemed to embrace every second of life.

About four years ago, however, Pete sensed that something began to change. Carmen was getting moodier. He tossed it off as having to do with menopause. She cut back on her volunteering. Within another two years, she'd elected to stop working and begin collecting the modest pension she'd accrued by working for the school system. Soon enough, she was sleeping more than ever. It made Pete wonder what she was doing so much of during that day that made her so tired by the time he got home.

One winter day, Carmen slipped on ice and took a fall down the steps of their house. The accident resulted in the major ligaments of her knee - the ACL (Anterior Cruciate Ligament) and the MCL (Medial Collateral Ligament) - being damaged. Due to the simultaneous tears to both ligaments, surgery was prescribed. Additionally, Carmen needed about four months of physical therapy (PT) to regain the best use of her knee.

Carmen was prescribed a rigorous PT regimen three times per week. With her not driving much, Pete tried to take her to as many appointments as he could.

Given the climate at work, however, he was a little afraid of keep taking time off to get Carmen to her appointments. Those kids at the office, it seemed, were breathing down his neck, just waiting for him to slip up so they could take over his accounts. He could feel the heat as younger co-workers dealt with him on a daily basis. He'd lost his mantle as "The Answer Man" and was now seen simply as "The *Old* Man."

Pete and his wife's three kids had all made it through college on money saved mostly through Pete's job. He had taken out a few tuition loans, but most had been paid back by now. Although he felt it was his duty and obligation to put all three children through college, Pete saw the process as backbreaking. When they were all finished, each of his kids took a job in a different part of the country.

Without the kids around to share some of the responsibilities of getting Carmen to her appointments, he had relied on the kindness of neighbors and local car service. Nonetheless, Pete felt a real pang of guilt each time he thought about his wife getting to PT without his help. There was just nothing he could do about it, he thought.

After finishing work for the day, Pete entered what seemed like an empty house. Carmen was home when he got there, but she no longer greeted him at the door, or from the kitchen table, or from the couch in the living room. She might call hello from upstairs or say nothing at all because she'd be asleep with the TV on. These days, there were a few home-cooked meals for Pete. He could rustle up a few things for himself, but he could never match his wife's kitchen skills. His versions of salami and scrambled eggs or macaroni and cheese from a box didn't match the flair of Carmen's lasagna, pork chops, or pan-seared salmon. More often than not, he found himself dialing up the local Chinese take-out place. When they recognized his voice, they often responded with, "Number four with fried rice?"

Signature Scene: The Quiet of the Kitchen

By the time Pete pulled into his driveway, the day had already calcified in his shoulders. He shut off the engine and sat for a moment in the dark, watching the porch light throw a pale triangle across the lawn. Inside, the house was warm. Inside, it was also quiet in a way that made him feel like an intruder.

He let himself in and listened - no television, no music, no footsteps meeting his at the door. Carmen was home; he could tell by the faint glow under the bedroom door upstairs. But she no longer moved toward him the way she used to. The silence felt personal, as if the rooms were keeping score.

In the kitchen, he loosened his tie and set his briefcase down with the careful precision of someone trying not to make noise. The refrigerator hummed. A clock ticked. On the counter, an old school photo of the kids - smiling, younger, still in need of him - leaned against the fruit bowl. Pete stared at it as if it were evidence from another life.

He opened the liquor cabinet like it was a tool drawer. One bottle became two. He told himself the same sentence he'd used for years - *just one to take the edge off* - and felt his body relax before the glass was even full. Anticipation did that now: relief arriving early, like a promise that kept getting easier to believe.

The first sip warmed his throat and softened the hard corners of the day. For a minute, he could breathe. Then the warmth thinned, and the familiar urge rose up behind it: make the quiet quieter. Make the worry smaller. Make tomorrow less sharp. Pete watched his own hand tip the bottle again and hated how automatic it felt.

Upstairs, a floorboard creaked. Pete froze with the glass half raised. He waited for Carmen to call down, to ask how his day was, to ask why he sounded like he was hiding something. Nothing came. The house stayed still. He set the glass behind the sink, as if that could hide the truth from both of them, and wondered when he had become a man who could solve anyone else's problems and still have no answer at home.

The Business Dinner Downfall

As things became more competitive at work, it seemed like the clients with whom he once had a commanding presence were becoming more demanding. People didn't want to be schmoozed during the day anymore. The day was for "working." These younger executives, who'd taken over from guys Pete had known for years, wanted to talk over dinner. They must have figured they could fit in guys like Pete between the time they left the office and were ready to take the train home. They could snag a free meal and be on their way.

He now regularly found himself driving into the city, against the grain of commuter traffic, to meet with a client at a steak place around the corner from Grand Central Station or Penn Station. At least the food was good.

At these dinners, Pete found that a lot of guys would go for the harder stuff when drinking. Why did it matter to Mr. Purchasing Manager what he drank or how much he had when any buzz he'd acquired during dinner would wear off on the train ride home?

For Pete, however, drinking with clients at dinner now took on a whole new dimension.

Pete had been a casual drinker for most of his life. A beer after playing softball; occasional wine with dinner; a martini when out with friends; maybe a couple of gin and tonic at a wedding. Getting a few drinks while away on business at a convention was never a big deal, and a cocktail with clients didn't seem to impair him. He'd always been able to get up and go to work in the morning, attend a seminar for the day, or take care of the family.

He was always involved with his kids - be it coaching little league, watching karate demonstrations, or driving the youngest to dance classes. Among families in the neighborhood or people he'd coached with, he was never characterized as a drinker. He usually had only two beers at the Memorial Day or Labor Day picnics. In all this, Pete couldn't remember a time when he felt sloppy, out of control, or incapable of doing what he was supposed to do.

Lately, though, when he met with clients for dinner, there was a nagging feeling in his stomach. Pete took it as a sure sign that he was staring at oblivion. He had this feeling that each person he was wining and dining really wanted to deal with someone younger, someone slicker. Someone who also spent half his time monitoring a BlackBerry for text messages, e-mails, and stock quotes - like they did.

Now, after all those years talking to clients, he faced every dinner meeting with a nervous stomach. And the only way that sick feeling seemed to go away was after his second drink.

These dinners with clients had shifted Pete's alcohol

preference to two kinds of drinks: the whiskey sour and the Brandy Alexander.

Both drinks conjured up images of sophistication for him.

During his childhood, Pete had seen relatives at weddings and fancy dinners saunter up to the bar and request both. He especially remembered Uncle Doug asking for a whiskey sour. Uncle Doug; the guy he rarely saw without a suit on, the guy who drove the latest-model sporty convertible, the guy who bought him the coolest stuff on each birthday. It was Uncle Doug who let Pete try his first whiskey sour.

These traditional drinks, unspoiled by time, tasted just right. The whiskey sour was satisfying with its sweet lemon accents. The Brandy Alexander hit the spot with its complex fruit flavor accented by dark crème de cacao. They were smooth going down and provided warmth exactly where it was needed.

After Pete's second drink, that feeling in his stomach would subside. After his third drink, he'd feel like he could talk to clients without fear. He didn't need to feel out what kind of guy he was dealing with - Ivy grad or Joe Six-pack; whatever they drank was no longer his concern. He'd feel powerful again; like time didn't matter, like he was back to being "The Answer Man."

For a while, it seemed, business got better after Pete had settled into his routine of whiskey sours and Brandy Alexanders. The spike in sales had added to his confidence, and he vowed to keep it up.

"If it ain't broke, don't fix it," he'd say.

A few months after starting this routine, however, three-drink nights turned into four and five-drink nights. It seemed that the nervous feeling in his stomach needed three drinks just to be kept at bay. Pete was finding ways to get to the restaurant early so he could down two drinks before seeing a client. When he was ordering what appeared to be his second or third drinks with dinner, the client didn't know Pete was already on his fourth or fifth of the night.

As things progressed, Pete expanded his drinking routine. He'd have between two and five drinks with dinner, but once the client's contact was signed, he'd put on his coat and bid his dinner companion farewell. Since he usually parked at a lot in the opposite direction of Grand Central Station or Penn Station, it looked to the client like Pete was just heading to his car.

But then, Pete would double back to the bar in the restaurant and order another whiskey sour or Brandy Alexander. Five drinks became more like six or seven.

What was the harm in what he was doing? Pete figured. He was getting more business, he was getting home at a reasonable hour, he never had trouble driving, and his wife never wondered what he was doing.

"Who knows," Pete thought, "maybe she's having an affair anyway. That must be tiring her out at least a little." And by the time he got home, he knew she'd already be asleep.

Professor Pete, Master Mixologist

Nights without client meetings were something that Pete usually looked forward to. He faced none of the hassles of driving through the Lincoln Tunnel. He could check in on Carmen and maybe catch some baseball on TV.

But these nights were starting to feel kind of dull. Not that Pete was an overly competitive guy, but at home, nothing was on the line. That feeling of fighting for his very existence - like when he took on a client - just wasn't there.

Pete often used his time at home to watch his favorite baseball team play from the comfort of his living room. But one night, it just hit him like an inside pitch aimed straight at the noggin - that smell of a whiskey sour.

He could feel it on his lips, hitting his taste buds, traveling down his throat, and hitting his nervous stomach with a warm blanket of assurance. He had a bottle of whiskey in the house, but not the drink mix.

He would soon fix that. A short trip to the liquor store yielded two packs of whiskey sour mix, another bottle of whiskey, and a bottle of brandy. Pete brought everything into the kitchen, where he became "Professor Pete, Master Mixologist."

He sat in front of the TV and thought, what's wrong with a whiskey sour and a baseball game? And with the season his team was having (one that would ultimately end in colossal failure and would knock them out of the playoffs) a whiskey sour was more like a necessity.

At work the next day, Pete thought that making his own Brandy Alexander that night would be nice. He had looked up a recipe on the Web that sounded easy enough.

1 ½ ounces brandy

1 ounce dark crème de cacao

1 ounce half-and-half

¼ teaspoon grated nutmeg

He had the brandy, knew there was some half-and-half in the fridge, and figured there was a tin of nutmeg in that lazy Susan where Carmen kept the spices. But crème de cacao?

That would require another trip to the liquor store on the way home.

On those days at home, Pete would switch his "master mixologist" persona between whiskey sour expert and Brandy Alexander connoisseur. In the case of both drinks, he'd find ways to maximize alcohol use without drowning any flavor. He could stretch the amount of brandy from 1½ to 2 ounces, and the measurement of whiskey from 2 to 3 ounces.

What is Going On in Pete's Brain?

For some people, alcoholism starts as a response to stress, and that stress can trigger alcoholism at any point in life. People with alcohol use disorder use drinking to generate a "good" feeling - also called euphoria or a "high." They get that high when alcohol helps increase the release of dopamine, a chemical in the brain categorized as a neurotransmitter, which acts as a messenger from one nerve cell to another.

Dopamine, in fact, helps guide most of the choices that people make every day. A person is always deciding what is rewarding and what is painful - we all weigh those choices against the benefits of long-term rewards and long-term pain. But in the case of the alcoholic's brain, even the anticipation of alcohol helps raise dopamine levels, and it makes an alcoholic want to drink even more.

As the production of dopamine molecules rises, receptors in Pete's brain rush to read them. This helps stimulate his brain's "reward" system. A reward is sought following a reaction that is triggered in the brain's cortico-mesolimbic system - the place that governs emotions.

Three structures in the limbic system are crucial elements

in producing pleasure and, ultimately, alcohol use disorder. They are:

The , which forms the basis of our memories. It preserves recollections associated with drinking alcohol. Such "positive" memories can include minute details about the environment in which he drinks.

The *amygdala*, which helps decode emotions and stimuli that seem threatening. Many of our body's "alarm" circuits are in the amygdala. Ultimately, it provides a person with perceptions that are either pleasurable or disagreeable.

The , or *insula*, which may play a role in the way people consciously seek pleasure from food, alcohol, or drugs.

Pete's hippocampus can remember everything about the experience of drinking alcohol with extreme clarity. It will capture the "high." It will also retain the people, places, objects, smells, and tastes associated with the drive that triggered his desire to drink. At the same time, his amygdala goes into overdrive, producing a strong, 'agreeable' response. So, when Pete experiences even some of the elements associated with drinking, the hippocampus triggers the production of dopamine by firing off another neurotransmitter, glutamate. Glutamate, which is also involved in the process of long-term memory, helps Pete's brain receive a signal that he is about to experience something good. Thus, thoughts immediately surface about alcohol, and they're accompanied by very strong emotional urges to drink.

As time goes by, the cortico-mesolimbic system can become progressively more demanding before it produces a response. That's because alcohol can damage the system and other parts of the brain. Damage to these areas creates an imbalance between neurotransmitters (like dopamine) and their receptors. Meaning the brain's ability to interpret and respond to the information carried by the neurotransmitter dopamine becomes weaker. It essentially starts to ask for more information, and the only way to produce more information is to drink more alcohol.

Because he is alcohol dependent, when Pete drinks, the alcohol causes a short circuit in the brain. Incorrect signals are sent out; they tell the body something is good when it's not, or bad when it's really good.

Taking One for the Team

As the baseball season progressed, his favorite team became involved in a tight pennant race. These guys had been one strike away from playing in the league championship series last year and were expected to run away with the division this year. They were in command of first place for most of the season, but now they were watching their dreaded rival creep up in the rearview mirror.

Pete's "boys of summer" had a seven-game lead on September 12 but were about to enter a collapse of historic proportions.

September 14: A 3-2 loss to hated rivals in 10 innings at home; it took four whiskey sours to get through that game, three of which Pete downed after the fifth innings.

September 15: A 5-3 loss; three Brandy Alexanders.

September 17: A 12-4 loss to a much worse team. Pete spent the night with a client. He had five drinks, two before dinner, two during, and one more at the bar afterward, where he caught the disappointing 8th and 9th innings.

September 18: A 9-8 loss.

The next match, tipsily figuring he could change their luck, Pete began the game with a beer. In the fifth inning, with his guys holding a 7-3 lead, the starting pitcher fell apart. The opposition scored six unanswered runs. In an effort to shift the score, Pete switched back to whiskey sours.

On Sunday, September 23, his boys struggled to a 7-6 win in 11 innings. Pete drank moderately during the first 8 innings, two whiskey sours over the course of about three hours, but he downed three more between the 9th and 11th. His brother-in-law, Ted, came over for Sunday dinner and decided to watch the game beforehand. He was there to hear Pete's tirade when the game was over.

"I can't believe it!" he yelled. "We play a team that's mediocre at best, and we gotta go 11 innings to put 'em down. You know what the problem is? We're paying millions for a guy who never does anything in the clutch. One scratch on his knee and he goes down like a ton of bricks."

"Pete, the guy ran into a wall trying to stop another run from scoring," Ted said. "What more do you want from him?"

"Are you kidding?" Pete snapped. "He's supposed to do that! You don't see me begging out of paying for you when you come over here and eat dinner and drink my liquor!"

Pete and Ted never had any major disagreements over the years, so this one came as a real doozy.

"What are you talking about?" asked Ted.

"I'm saying that guy has no heart whatsoever, and neither do you, ya flakey bandwagon fan!"

Pete was shouting. Carmen came out of the kitchen.

"Pete, calm down!" Carmen pleaded. "It's just a game!"

"It's not just a game...it's more than that," he retorted. "I'm sick and tired of feeding this mooch every Sunday, only to find out he knows nothing about baseball!"

"Listen, Pete," Ted broke in, "just because your team's playing some bad ball is no reason to take it out on me. I can take your trash-talking, but where's this attack coming from?"

"Oh, what do you know, bandwagon boy!" Pete shot back.

Ted had heard enough.

"You know what, Pete? You've got a problem. And I think it has to do with your drinking. You think I don't notice how many whiskey sours you had during the game?"

"It's none of your goddamn business what I'm drinking or how much I've had!"

With that, Ted started walking toward the door.

"Pete, you need help! I'll be back when you've sobered up! Carmen, you know how to reach me."

Later, during dinner, Carmen decided it was time to say something to Pete.

"You know, you think I don't notice that something's different about you," she said. "But you've got something going on. I see the bottles in the closet. I mean, we always had some liquor around the house for guests, but never anything like..."

"I'm fine," he interrupted. "I like to have that stuff around because I enjoy it, and it's cheaper than going to a bar."

"Pete, I'm not so sure you're fine," she said. "You and Teddy never argued like that before. And over something so stupid. It's like something is taking over you."

"What, you think I can't hold my liquor?"

"I don't care if you can hold anything!" she said. "I just

need to know you're taking care of yourself and me, and that you're not too proud to stop acting like a jackass."

"I'm fine," he said. "Maybe I had a little too much today, and I'm angry with how the season's going. I'll call Ted during the week."

"Pete, I'm not so sure this is about baseball," she said. "I've been getting calls from the bank. They say we've missed the last two mortgage payments. How can that be?"

"I gotta check that out," he said. "Maybe I forgot to send a check, or they just didn't get it."

"But Pete, that's never been a problem for us in the past, even when we were making less money."

Carmen was building up to this moment in her mind but had trouble getting out the words. No better time than the present, she thought.

"Pete, I think you should talk to somebody," she said. "I think you might need help. Maybe you should call the guys at AA and find some things out."

"What, have you been talking to people down at the church again?" he screamed. "One conversation, and you're a goddamn expert. I'm not talking to anyone at AA! Talk about a bunch of whiners. They like to share in each other's misery. Why would I want to be around those people?"

Noticing her flinch, Pete backed off, but only slightly.

"Maybe I need to cut back a little, that's all," he said. "But, I'm fine."

Later that night, after Carmen went to bed, Pete drank a little more. He was just nursing a few, after all.

Pete was "The Answer Man." He knew how to handle his liquor - and his problems.

Running Out of Answers

The next morning, Pete didn't wake up until 11 a.m. Carmen had caught a ride with a neighbor to one of her PT appointments. There was a message on his answering machine from his department's administrative assistant.

"Pete, this is Julie Brand. Mark Hughes asked me to give you a call to see what was up. When you get a chance, please call me. Thanks."

Pete's head hurt. He was usually able to make things go away with three aspirin and a 16-ounce coffee. Today, he wasn't so sure that that was going to do the trick.

He cleared his throat about 10 times and rehearsed speaking in his clearest voice before finally making the call.

"Julie, this is Pete. Tell Mark I'm not feeling so great, and I'm staying home today."

"Okay, I'll let him know," Julie said. "But he also wanted me to mention that your sales reports are due in by tomorrow."

Great, Pete thought, muttering assent and ending the call.

Throughout mid-June, he had been riding high with new and repeat sales. But things had dropped off quite a bit lately. He'd managed to avoid submitting reports for the last two months, but now he knew that he might have to face the truth.

A few days later, Pete had a meeting with Mark Hughes, the company's vice president of sales development.

"So Pete," Hughes began, "You've been a leading guy around here for quite some time. But I'm looking at your sales reports, and it seems that you're down about 35 percent since July. So...what gives?"

"Just a little slump, Mark," Pete answered smoothly. "You

know, spending drops off in the summer and the economy hasn't been great. I'm sure I'll get my numbers back up before year's end, with all that end-of-fiscal-year spending."

"Well, that would be great," Hughes said. "Listen, I want to make sure you have everything you need at your disposal to make that happen. I also want to know if you're feeling okay. Not that I'm in such great shape myself, but you look a little more tired than usual."

"Oh, you know," said Pete. "Carmen's had a lot of physical therapy and doctors' appointments lately. I guess I've just had a lot going on."

Excuses had never been his thing. Even in rough economies, he'd still been a top sales guy. He used spreadsheets to work out lease terms with clients and to figure out the next great product to fit their needs.

Whew, that was close, thought Pete. He figured no one had really noticed anything different about him. It turned out that wasn't the case.

Work Hard, Play Hard

He knew he needed things to pick up. Maybe the client meeting he had tonight would help. Pete was scheduled to meet with the logistics manager from a web company, one of the big ones that had survived the dot-com bomb of the late nineties and was now sitting on top of the world. These kinds of guys were always touting how they found "new ways to work", and in Pete's mind, that meant new office floor configurations. What a perfect way to get in there and let them know about his company's furniture and ergonomic solutions.

Instead of a visit to the steakhouse around the corner from

Penn Station, he was taking this guy on top of Penn Station, to Madison Square Garden, for a basketball game. He'd snagged box seats near midcourt and passed to one of the arena's private clubs upstairs. He'd be meeting the guy on the steps into the Garden, so they could go in together.

On his way over, he felt that nagging, pre-client-meeting feeling in his stomach. So he stopped off at a bar around the corner before getting to the Garden.

The web company's logistics manager was a 28-year-old named James. Smart guy, top-flight MBA degree, and someone who had a direct link to the venture capital guys that were using the web company as its latest cash cow. And, as he learned later, was also part of a new generation of execs who lived by the motto "work hard, play hard."

First, they went up to The Club Bar & Grill in the Garden. Like the site said, "If you want the best in fine dining, exemplary service, and elegant ambiance," The Club is for you.

Pete ordered a Brandy Alexander. James had bourbon on the rocks.

By the time dinner came, Pete was on what looked like his second but was really his fourth drink. James was just starting his second. That fourth one seemed to be giving Pete more confidence than he'd anticipated. He started telling stories about the history of office furniture - the development of the workstation, the invention of the rotating chair, the genius of the tilting keyboard hutch. Such stories were not usually part of Pete's repertoire, but tonight they were just flying from his mouth. And he had no idea whether James really gave two hoots.

The duo finished their dinner with a digestif, the kind of drink that's supposed to aid your digestion. James apparently knew a bit about sherry, so Pete followed his lead. Then it was time to take their seats about 10 rows from center court.

During the game's first time-out, James motioned to the waitress who was taking orders for their section of luxury seats. He asked her for a beer, and Pete followed his lead. This ritual happened again in the second quarter, at halftime, and in the third quarter. By the start of the fourth, Pete was completely hammered.

The game was tight, and with 10:32 left in the fourth, one of the home team's players was fouled hard as he was attempting a layup. The opposing player was assessed with a personal foul but not a technical foul.

This decision infuriated Pete. He felt something building up inside him; it was rage.

While the rest of the crowd merely booed, Pete screamed obscenities at the ref. He was standing on the top of his chair, shouting. He had no idea that the entire arena was watching him.

Within 30 seconds, six guards surrounded Pete.

He started yelling.

"What? Can't a guy get mad at a bad call?" This he followed up with, "Jeez, you're breakin' my arm!"

His dinner companion, the hard-working, hard-playing James, stood in horror as Pete was led away. A few cups of soda rained down from the upper deck toward Pete and his new law enforcement friends. James slowly sat back in his seat, with a pained expression best captured by the words, "I'm not really with that guy."

Within 20 minutes, two guards escorted Pete out onto Seventh Avenue in front of Penn Station. Shortly after the men returned inside, Pete made his way through the departing crowd across Seventh Avenue to 31st Street. He found a dark corner and began to vomit his brains out.

Though he had driven his car into the city, Pete couldn't remember the garage he'd parked in. Was it on 29th, or was it the one near the Post Office? Not knowing exactly where his car was located probably acted as the only deterrent to his driving home. Pete figured once he'd thrown up, he was "shocked" into a state of sobriety. But without his car, he felt forced to take a train from Penn Station and call a cab once he'd arrived at the station closest to home.

We Need to Talk

The next day, Pete didn't wake up until almost noon. Again, there was a message on his machine from Julie Brand, his department's administrative assistant.

"Hi Pete, this is Julie Brand. Mr. Hughes missed you in the office this morning and was wondering where you are. He wants to speak with you as soon as possible, so give me a call when you get this message."

"Oh no," was the only thing he could mutter. Just two words, yet saying them sent shockwaves through his brain and made his head feel like a spike was being driven into his cerebral cortex.

At about 12:30, after a 20-minute shower, four aspirins, and a double shot of antacid, Pete built up enough strength to call Julie and get on the phone with Hughes.

"Pete," sighed Hughes, "I spoke with James from that web company you were trying to sign. He said you stood on your seat, screaming obscenities at the top of your lungs before security threw you out on your ass."

"Does that mean I didn't get the account?" Pete asked sarcastically.

"Are you kidding me?" Hughes shot back. "He said he wouldn't do business with us in a million years! Make sure you're in here first thing tomorrow morning. We need to talk."

Pete was in Mark Hughes' office by 9 a.m. Wednesday, wearing what he thought was his best, wrinkle-free suit (although he couldn't remember the last time it had been dry-cleaned).

"Pete, you know I've been one of your biggest fans for a long time," Hughes said. "We've been together for 12 years. Now, I'm not exactly sure what you're going through, but I've got a pretty good idea.

"The thing is," Hughes continued, exhaling, "it's my job to make sure that you're able to do the best job you can. So this is what I'm strongly suggesting. See this brochure? It's from our employee assistance program, the EAP. They've got people you can talk to and figure out whether you need to make some kind of change.

"Look, whatever it takes and whatever you decide to do, I'm with you, Pete," Hughes said. "You've been here too long for me to sit here and pretend like nothing's wrong. We need you old guys to show everyone how it's done. So, take a look at this material, give these people a call, and let me know what you decide to do."

Pete wasn't so sure that he had as big a problem as Hughes was making it out to be. Still, if nothing else, he figured he needed the paycheck.

The AUDIT

A few days later, a counselor from the company's EAP gave Pete the name of a physician who had experience in treating addiction. An initial consultation with a doctor and two sessions of counseling would be covered. After that, Pete would have to rely on the company's insurance for any detox sessions or rehab stays.

The doctor gave Pete a complete physical. He found that Pete's blood pressure was up. Also, Pete's weight was 20 pounds higher than he could ever remember. Most importantly, the doctor administered the Alcohol Use Disorders Identification Test (AUDIT).

AUDIT, which was developed by the World Health Organization, screens people for at-risk drinking and dependence (heavy drinking). The test scores 10 questions on a scale of 1 to 4. If the total score is three or less, it means a person's drinking does not exceed the limits for healthy adults. A score between 4 and 7 indicates that a person may need to cut down or quit drinking. Scores above 8 indicate that unhealthy alcohol use is occurring. Anything 16 or above means professional help is a must.

Pete's score was 22.

The doctor recommended three rehab centers, and two of them were in Pete's insurance plan. Both were within an hour's drive of home. Pete found out that his insurance would cover a seven-day period of detox and 28 days of in-house treatment.

Pete looked at the online page for each facility. Both places seemed purely pastoral. Rolling hills, swimming pools, nicely appointed bedrooms. They had their similarities. Both:

Offered detox and rehab at the same site.

Employed the Minnesota Model of recovery, which embraced the 12-step program endorsed by AA.

Said they had excellent cognitive-behavioral therapy (CBT) programs. CBT, sometimes called "talk therapy," is designed to help people become more aware of their triggers for drinking and gain a better understanding of themselves.

Were certified by the two major organizations that monitor rehab facilities, the Commission on Accreditation of Rehabilitation Facilities (CARF), and the Joint Commission.

As for advantages, one offered massages, and the other said it had an outstanding series of live lectures and interactive programs.

He really needed recommendations on both places, but people around him didn't talk about rehab facilities, and he wasn't about to go seeking the opinion of friends and relatives, especially his kids. The problem was that neither he nor Carmen could find a site or other information source that had definitive standards measuring the effectiveness of rehab programs.

Pete rolled the dice and went with Sobriety House. This facility touted its excellent live lecture program. He'd always enjoyed attending seminars as part of his job, so he figured it wouldn't be so bad to listen to a new person every day.

Taking the First Step

Detox was no picnic - lots of sweats, shakes, hallucinations, and vomiting. Pete couldn't even wear his own clothes; he had to stay in pajamas issued by Sobriety House. All his personal belongings, including his wallet with pictures of Carmen and the kids, were stowed away for "safekeeping."

He couldn't just go shave in the morning. He had to go to the nurses' station and ask for his razor and shaving cream. When he was done, he had to give them back. He wasn't allowed to call Carmen for the first three days, and when he was finally allowed to talk to her, he had to ask permission, and the number had to be dialed for him. All conversations had to occur in the open, where at least one side could be heard. Pete started to feel better on his fifth day there.

By day seven, he began the Sobriety House residential program, which included weekday schedules that were even tighter than work. He attended lectures that described the details of addiction and went to group counseling. He was assigned a personal counselor whose one-on-one sessions were supplemented with group meetings each morning and afternoon.

The group meetings were designed for everyone to explore their problems, feelings, changes, and conflicts that arose during treatment. During meetings, he got to hear stories about Marie, the accountant, Mike the stockbroker, and Chuck the pipefitter. Each of them seemed to reach a crisis point where they woke up naked in an alley, covered with vomit in the bed of a stranger, or in the emergency room clinging to life.

As part of the program, Pete was assigned a "buddy" who was a little farther along in the rehab process. His buddy was Sal, a guy who owned a body shop in Bayonne. This was Sal's third time in rehab.

Pete was introduced to the First Step process during treatment; the introduction to a 12 step program. His counselor initiated that step by reviewing Pete's history with alcohol, the effects that using it was having on his life, the impact it was having on the lives of those around him, and the negative consequences of drinking to excess. Pete was then asked to write an autobiography. This was meant to pinpoint what experiences he had with alcohol and to understand the triggers that made him want to put away seven Brandy Alexanders in three hours just about every night.

The one thing he did pick up by writing things out was an explanation for his outburst at the basketball game. That rage was the manifestation of self-pity. Pete acknowledged that he was feeling sorry for himself and that unlike in the past, he felt as though he couldn't solve his own problems. At least now, he felt like he was doing the right thing.

Since Sobriety House incorporated AA's 12-step process, there were constant reminders that he needed to give himself over to a higher power. Pete had never been a particularly religious man. In fact, he had drifted away from the Catholic Church, of which his parents were such fervent followers.

Sure, when his kids were young, they were enrolled in religious education and made their sacraments, just as Pete and Carmen had. To Pete, though, joining a church was just a way he could keep playing softball once in a while with the men's group. Carmen was more into Catholicism, and since she'd gotten breast cancer, her spirituality seemed to have risen up a notch.

Still, he spoke to the center's chaplain a few times, when other patients around him were doing it, which made it seem like the right thing to do. But he was never crazy about the outcome of these conversations. Each talk could be boiled down to the phrase: 'You're powerless over your situation. If you don't give yourself over to Jesus Christ, your chances of being healed are slim to none.'

The Fog Lifts

After 28 days, Pete was discharged. It was February in New Jersey, during one of those weeks that tempts people with the promise of spring when temperatures fluctuate between the '50s and '60s, and the sun always feels a little warmer. Like a little kid, Pete had the urge to toss off his coat and have a catch. On this day, his senses just seemed a little sharper. It was like that alcoholic fog had finally lifted.

Pete's brother-in-law, Ted, the same one with whom he'd had that heated argument, drove Carmen to Sobriety House to pick Pete up.

When they met him under the awning marking the Sobriety House entrance, Carmen popped out of the car. Pete gave her a huge hug, and they kissed. Both were in tears. Carmen looked better than he could remember.

"I'm sorry," was all he could say.

Then he gave Ted a big hug.

"Hey, Ted. I'm sorry," Pete said. "You're not a moocher."

Had he already started working AA's 12 steps? Wasn't this step nine? *Make direct amends with all persons we have harmed wherever possible, except when to do so would injure them or others.*

Pete had decided he would stay home for a week after rehab, to get re-acclimated to life without alcohol. He wanted to see how he would handle his time in a controlled environment, especially the afternoons and evenings when he was more prone to drink.

He also wanted to get into the habit of attending AA

meetings. Carmen had signed him up for a group that met nightly in the basement of their church. Pete also took an additional step in scouting out AA meetings in the city so he could catch meetings before entertaining clients or if he had to work late.

Pete gradually got back into the swing of things. At work, he had made an arrangement with Hughes to hold off on entertaining clients for a month. Once that period ended, his goal was to push for more lunch meetings. When his drinking was at its worst, he seemed to have no major problems at lunch; it was more like 2 p.m. when the craving for alcohol started knocking.

Things were going well. His plan for easing in at work was spot-on. That first month gave him the opportunity to reconnect with clients and figure out new ways to present data. Mark Hughes was happy to have him back. If he harbored any trace of bitterness, Hughes never seemed to show it.

Pete was going to daily AA meetings. He knew AA was something he had to stick with, but the meetings were tough. Every day it seemed like they were doing the same thing; opening with a prayer, sitting in a circle, and talking about the temptation of alcohol.

And new people kept showing up every other week to pour their souls out regarding how they'd gotten there. Pete was sympathetic to everyone, his story wasn't that different, but he didn't look forward to verbally reliving it.

Many times, the meetings resembled scenes from a bad Sunday morning televangelism show; replete with people shouting out, "Hallelujah!" and "Thank you, Jesus!" Some nights it was like people were playing a game called "Can You Top This?" Stories drifted from wild nights of drinking to waking up in a produce warehouse covered in star fruit and even having sex with toothless doormen on the condition of being rewarded with another mint julep. Not that Pete wanted to get completely away from thinking about recovery, but he was not a guy who dwelled too much on the past.

A Test of the Will

Four months sober.

It was time to start wooing new clients. And, inevitably, Pete was going to have to deal with the power brokers of some major companies; guys who only seemed to have time to talk at night when they weren't doing "real work." But he felt ready.

Before meeting clients, he made a point of scouting out restaurants that didn't have bars. He was hoping to avoid steakhouses because it seemed like the porterhouse always courted a strong alcoholic companion. But it wouldn't be long before he received an assignment that would test his will.

A big pharmaceutical client was expanding its operations in the city - something that was almost unheard of lately due to the soaring cost of Manhattan office space. The location's operations manager wanted to set up a dinner meeting to discuss how Pete's company could meet their needs. He insisted they meet at one of the city's best steakhouses, claiming he knew the Maître d' and half the staff.

Before that Wednesday night meeting, Pete made sure he could attend the AA group he'd scouted on East 46th Street. The meeting started at 6, and Pete figured he could catch most of it before heading to the client dinner on 53rd and

Lexington by 7. His hope was that the meeting would give him an extra shot of strength.

When he got to the steakhouse, the place smelled like heaven. The scent of finely prepared meat wafted through the air. He even could identify the smell of specially prepared sides - creamed spinach, the tomato and onion platter, and the beef barley soup. The place had a long bar of handcrafted teak that was polished to a smooth shine. By virtue of the fact that he arrived close to the appointment time, he would not have the chance to fall into his old habit of downing a few before the meeting.

Still, his stomach nagged him. That old feeling that he might be meeting his match was back.

He sat at a table by the window with Larry Green, the impeccably dressed 31-year-old ops manager. Larry had also brought along Phil Tobia, the assistant ops manager. Larry had joked that he owed Phil a steak after the Super Bowl, so he figured he'd kill two birds with one stone.

The waiter came around, handed each a menu, then asked the loaded question.

"Gentlemen, what can I start you off with to drink?"

Here we go, Pete thought.

Larry went first. "I'll have a whiskey sour."

Don't do this to me! Pete thought.

"I'll have the same," said Phil.

"Sir?" said the waiter as he turned toward Pete.

He was silent. How could he admit to them that he was an alcoholic and couldn't drink? This was like his first major test since rehab. What was he going to do?

He could *smell* the whiskey sour. And it smelled good. The

ingredients to make the drink were nowhere near the table, but it was like someone had connected a circuit from his brain to his nose. And before he could catch his tongue, the words came rolling out.

"Make it three!"

The Backslide

Pete had somehow managed to hold himself to two whiskey sours that night. He thought that maybe he'd experienced a momentary slip and would be able to recover with the help of AA.

But a week later, at another client meeting, he faced the same dilemma.

"I'll have a Brandy Alexander," he told the waiter.

Soon, Pete's drinking habits were back. What had taken him a few years to build up to the first time around was now back at full speed within a month. He was downing two drinks before client meetings, three or four during. He thought he wasn't babbling too much during meetings, but he could never be quite sure.

He thought he was a little smarter this time around since instead of driving to the city for client meetings, he was taking trains. He thought, "How messed up could I really be if I'm that far ahead of things?"

Within six months of finishing rehab, he was again waking up some days at 11 a.m., only to find messages from Julie Brand on his answering machine. He thought his sales numbers were fine, and because he'd only really started meeting clients about two months ago, he figured Hughes was still treating him with kid gloves.

He was back to arguing about stupid things. He was always

irritable. His team was playing up and down baseball, and the idea that they could face another season-ending collapse haunted him. He had stopped attending AA meetings, although he told Carmen he was there all the time.

All these red flags should have been enough for him to gather his thoughts and say it was time to get his life straight again. But the straw that broke the camel's back had nothing to do with work, arguing, or watching baseball.

Carmen was set to have a minor operation. All those times she was flopping into bed by 7, while Pete's alcoholic mind speculated that having taken a daytime lover was wearing her out, were actually linked to a thyroid problem. Her doctor said that removing her thyroid might help her gain some much-needed energy. She was scheduled to have the operation on a Thursday, stay in the hospital for observation overnight, and be picked up by Pete around 10:30 the next morning. Pete had made arrangements to take Thursday and Friday off to be with Carmen.

The operation went fine. Pete stayed in the hospital with Carmen and left when visiting hours were over at 8 p.m.

The whole day may have been stressful for Carmen, but it was killing Pete. He needed a drink.

He hit the liquor store on the way home. He needed a fresh supply of brandy, whiskey, and all the things needed to make his drinks.

By 10 p.m., he was into his third whiskey sour. By midnight, he'd had six.

Friday at noon, he heard the phone ringing. The answering machine picked up, and he could hear the message.

"This is Bernice Carroll at the discharge desk at St.

Luke's," said the voice. "Your wife, Carmen, was due to be discharged at 10:30, and she says you were supposed to come to pick her up. We've been keeping her in a room for as long as we can, and we've been calling you since 11. Please call us back as soon as possible. Thank you."

Oh my God, thought Pete.

There he was, feeling like a complete slug with a pounding headache, a mouth as dry as sandpaper, and dressed in the same clothes he had on the night before. The hospital was at least a half-hour away.

He threw on a new pair of pants and a shirt, brushed his teeth, and swallowed five aspirin in hopes that he'd be functional. The problem was, he felt like he'd been hit by a bus.

Pete hopped behind the wheel and started making his way toward Route 3.

The next thing he remembered was a policeman asking him if he was all right. He had wrapped the car around a fire hydrant. He was given a Breathalyzer test to determine his blood-alcohol level. He passed but ended up being cited for reckless driving.

All the while, Carmen was waiting for him at St. Luke's. Finally, at 1 p.m., she called her brother Ted at work and asked him to come pick her up.

Relapse

They say that relapse is part of recovery. In fact, of the people who *don't* partner medication with some type of psychosocial therapy (such as CBT, one-on-one meetings with a therapist, or group therapy), up to 70 percent will resume drinking within one year.

There are people who swear by AA and other 12-step groups, but there is no evidence that people in these programs are emotionally or spiritually superior to people who get clean and sober via other methods.

For proponents of these groups, it may be helpful for them to believe that theirs is the best way, but this can hurt people for whom AA doesn't work. The 12-step model can actually harm people who've relapsed, as those programs stipulate that once a person begins to slip, he or she is powerless to stop. Unfortunately, people with stronger beliefs in this perspective often face longer and more damaging relapses.

Beginning Again

This time, Pete chose the other rehab center that was recommended to him; Shady Acres, the one with the massages. He figured if the first one didn't work, maybe a change would help.

Shady Acres seemed to put an emphasis on couples and family therapy. Their literature said that family support is an important part of recovery and that involving a spouse in treatment could increase the chances of successful recovery. Carmen was still annoyed with him over his failure to pick her up at St. Luke's, but Pete knew she wanted him to get better.

Before entering Shady Acres, Pete called his kids to tell them that he was going back to rehab. Where last time he had wanted to shield them from ever knowing how badly he'd screwed up, this time he wanted their help to get him through things, and he hoped they could fly in to see him on a weekend.

One of the biggest differences this time around, however, was that his insurance would cover detox but not his entire stay in rehab. Pete was going to have to pay $14,000 out of his own pocket if he wanted to stay in the program.

Detox was much the same: shakes, chills, headaches, hallucinations. The residential program had its similarities to his first go-round at Sobriety House. Group therapy, counseling, writing things out. He was buddied up with a guy in his 30's after the first week. Now Pete was the "Sal" - the three-time offender who was Pete's buddy during the Sobriety House stint.

The massages were good.

Shady Acres was also big on exercise. Pete picked up riding a stationary bike. It made him sweat like he hadn't in 15 years. He figured, why not? He had all the time in the world.

Carmen came by on weekends; Ted drove her. Pete was always happy to see her, but every time he did, he felt like a failure. When he took that first drink back at the steakhouse with the guys from the pharmaceutical company, he knew he was doing something wrong. By the time he took another drink a few days later, he didn't care. It was like his willpower flew straight out the window, and his brain was on autopilot.

He found out from his counselor that some experts believe relapse is part of recovery. Some of those same experts say that the more times an alcoholic tried to stay sober, the greater his chances were of sustaining the success he'd achieved during treatment.

Great, Pete thought bleakly. That's probably in a perfect 'treatment world.' I bet none of them factored in how much money treatment was gonna cost once their insurance benefits ran out."

Feeling Obligated

When Pete finished up at Shady Acres, it was back to AA. He figured he'd stick with the one in the basement of the church, even though this second rehab stint made him more cynical than ever about the presence of an almighty God. "If he was so mighty, how come he didn't stop me from drinking in the first place," Pete thought.

Pete went to AA because it was one of those things he was told he *should* do. But his discomfort level with the program grew stronger.

Many individuals with alcohol use disorder who follow the Minnesota Model 12-step treatment programs, such as AA, fervently believe that their method is superior to all others. They often view with suspicion people who recover without attending meetings. And if those people had problems, it was attributed to a lack of AA-nurtured spiritual growth.

Worse still, fervent AA followers seem to perceive people who stop attending meetings as being in danger of relapse. People who stay sober for long periods without the program are called "dry drunks." They see these folks as having given up alcohol but not the negative personality traits that were the underlying reason for their alcoholism.

With fears like that eating at him, it was no wonder Pete kept up his AA routine. What haunted him most, though, was the thought of how he'd gone to a meeting just before getting together with the pharmaceutical clients, and it didn't provide enough momentum to help him say "no."

He wished there was another way.

Tempted

Hughes had been patient with Pete during his second rehab stint and subsequent return to work. Pete again asked for a period of time to stay in the office and get reacquainted with his clients and the data that supported his sales efforts. When he was ready to go back into the field, however, some of his best clients had been given to other sales reps.

He wasn't happy with the decision, especially because his income had already suffered over the last year due to rehab stints. But he figured he had made it through hard times before and would do so again.

As could be expected, about four months later, Pete was facing the prospect of getting out of his daytime comfort zone for entertaining clients. Another year older and closer to retirement, Pete knew he had to figure out a way to return to form and run with the big boys.

His first nighttime client dinner was with the director of purchasing for one of the nation's largest mobile phone operators. He knew that even a small contract could mean a huge payday. The purchasing manager insisted that they meet at one of the city's best Japanese restaurants. The kind of place where they cook at your table and the saké flows freely.

When he got there, the purchasing director ordered a Japanese beer - a Sapporo. Then, the waiter turned to Pete. "Can I get you anything, sir?"

Pete paused. He'd rehearsed this in his mind a thousand times.

"Club soda and lime," he said.

On the inside, Pete felt a sense of victory, but he was also nervous. In fact, as the purchasing director ordered a second and third Sapporo, Pete could sense the barley and hops making their way toward his nose. Beer was not his drink of choice, but the idea of getting some alcohol in his system seemed, well...intoxicating.

Pete had managed to make it through the meeting. It went well. The new business looked promising. But he also had a nagging sense that he'd be tempted again and again. How would he handle it next time?

Hope on the Horizon

A few days later, Pete visited a family physician. He'd gotten the name of Dr. Ben Stewart from Ted, who'd been his patient for years. His reason for going had nothing to do with alcohol - he was experiencing pain in his right shoulder every time he lifted his arm above his chest.

Like many men his age, Pete didn't go to the doctor too often. His aversion to them was part of an old school philosophy; there was no reason to see one unless something was really wrong.

As with any patient who was new to a practice, Pete was asked to fill out paperwork. Pete gave the standard information; birth date, height, weight, family history, other medical conditions, the reason for the visit.

There was also a question that asked: Have you had a problem with alcohol over the past five years? If so, explain.

Pete checked the 'yes' box. He wrote down that he had been in rehab twice over the past year.

As a new patient, Pete was given a routine physical. Dr. Stewart then felt Pete's shoulder and asked him what kind of problems he was having.

"Might be a slight rotator cuff tear," Dr. Stewart said. "This is pretty common in guys your age. It may have been triggered by some kind of trauma a while back, but it probably didn't begin to hurt until it had some time to get irritated. Do you recall having some kind of fall or another incident that may have put some impact on that shoulder?"

"Uh, I had a car accident about seven months ago," Pete said.

He didn't want to say much more than that.

"It might be a good idea to get you an MRI and see what's going on in there," Dr. Stewart said. "If it's minor, you might be recommended a cortisone shot and then do a few sessions of physical therapy. Let me get a few things together for you, and I'll be back in a minute."

Dr. Stewart came back, holding the paperwork that Pete had filled out earlier.

"Listen, Pete," he said. "I was looking at what you filled out earlier. I don't want to come off as being too threatening or anything like that, but I noticed you mentioned that you have a history of alcohol use disorder."

"Yep," Pete replied. "Two stints in rehab over the past year or so. It's been rough."

"So, how are you doing with everything now?" Dr. Stewart asked.

"Not bad," his patient answered sheepishly. "I'm keeping up with AA meetings and have been sober for about six months or so. But I'm back to entertaining clients. It's a big part of my job, and the temptation is really strong sometimes. A few days ago, I was with a guy, and he ordered a beer. Beer was never really my drink, but for some reason, it was calling out to me. It was like a kid with candy. I'm just not sure how I'm going to handle it next time."

"You know that's pretty common with people who have

alcohol problems," Dr. Stewart said. "Something in your brain is just not working right. Alcoholism is a chronic and relapsing brain disease. It changes the way your brain works. The good thing is that it is treatable."

"Medically treatable?" Pete asked.

"Yes," said Dr. Stewart. "There are some great medicines that have been out there for a while that are helping people stay sober."

It was like a light went on in Pete's head. Everyone seemed to tell him that the reason he couldn't refuse a drink was because his willpower was weak. The AA people were sending him the message that he hadn't completely turned himself over to a higher power. It all made him feel like a failure.

And even though he knew what drinking could do to his life, there were times that he felt like chucking it all and picking up a Brandy Alexander to calm everything down.

Nor was he alone. About 30 percent of Americans drink enough to be considered at risk for health and mental problems. Most doctors have trouble recognizing patients who need help. And only about 10 percent of patients with alcohol use disorder ever get quality treatment, according to the National Institute on Alcohol Abuse and Alcoholism (NIAAA).

But Pete was lucky to have seen Dr. Stewart. The doctor had recently read the NIAAA publication *Helping Patients Who Drink Too Much: A Clinician's Guide*. Dr. Stewart had also learned about the availability of alcohol recovery drugs that he could administer.

Did Pete Really Need Another Rehab Stint to Get Better?

"Pete, you ever heard of a drug called naltrexone or Vivitrol?" asked Dr. Stewart.

"I think I've heard about it," Pete answered. "But I don't know. The people at both rehabs and in AA say taking drugs to stop drinking is just a crutch. Some told me that instead of being addicted to alcohol, I'd end up being addicted to those drugs."

"That's one of those myths," Dr. Stewart said. "The drugs don't work like that. You don't end up addicted to them, and they don't have major side effects."

Naltrexone, which gained approval from the U.S. Food and Drug Administration (FDA) in 1994, was the first new alcohol cessation drug approved in about 50 years. Naltrexone works by reducing the desire for alcohol. It interferes with the part of the brain that produces the pleasure people get from drinking. In pill form, it is also known by the brand names ReViaTM and DepadeTM.

Vivitrol is the injectable form of naltrexone. Approved by the FDA in 2006, Vivitrol can be given once per month. What makes it so effective is that it controls alcohol cravings and nearly eliminates "slips" that can lead to full-blown relapses. It plugs into the opioid receptors in certain brain cells; opioids being substances produced in the body that produce a feeling of well-being (euphoria) and able to cause mood changes and cloudy thinking. Opioid receptors accept opioids and then relay their effects to other parts of the brain.

With the high from alcohol blocked by Vivitrol, the first drink that a person may be tempted to have is usually the last. Additionally, since alcoholics often realize when they're teetering on the brink of relapse, they are more apt to call someone for support before things get out of hand.

There is a myth that using drugs to recover from alcohol use disorder means a person is trading alcoholism for drug dependence. But people on whom these drugs were tested did not develop a tolerance for or dependence on the medication. Additionally, there is another myth - often propagated by people who fear all alcohol recovery drugs - that Vivitrol will interfere with the parts of their brain responsible for all types of pleasure. But Vivitrol actually works only on the opioid receptors that are connected with an alcohol high.

Embracing Stability

"Sign me up!" Pete told Dr. Stewart enthusiastically.

Pete knew it wasn't going to entirely replace the need for counseling and support, but he also thought it would give him the stability he needed to continue his life.

Getting the shot also proved to be the impetus for Pete to find support groups that provided an alternative to AA. He found a chapter of SOS (Secular Organizations for Sobriety) not far from his home.

He liked the fact that the group's philosophy differed from AA. SOS is an alternative recovery method for the treatment of patients with alcohol use disorder who are uncomfortable with the spiritual content of most 12-step programs. The group maintains that sobriety is separate from religion or spirituality and credits the individual for achieving and maintaining sobriety without reliance on a "higher power."

Unlike AA, which saw abstinence as the only path to recovery, SOS says it respects recovery in any form regardless of the path by which it is achieved. Pete liked the fact that SOS supports healthy skepticism about AA and encourages the understanding of alcohol use disorder through science. He also found it extremely helpful that he could connect with local and national members of his group through online meetings, chat rooms, and forums. That meant if he missed a meeting, it wouldn't feel like the end of the world.

Meeting Challenges

Within two weeks of receiving his first Vivitrol shot, Pete felt like his alcohol cravings had all but disappeared. But after six weeks, he was scheduled to meet a client for dinner. The meeting was to be at one of the steakhouses Pete used to frequent when his drinking was at its worst.

The challenges of his past came calling. The client ordered bourbon. Pete ordered a whiskey sour.

But halfway through his whiskey sour, *he put it down*. He just didn't feel like finishing it.

He made it through the client meeting without wanting another drink. It was a real breakthrough. Suddenly, he didn't feel like he had to mimic a client to get the client's business.

When he got home, he joined an SOS chat room and talked about what had happened to him. He found the support he needed, went to bed at a reasonable hour, and, more importantly, woke up the next day and got to work on time.

Rehab Stints, Endless Counseling, Life Savings Lost... or Vivitrol?

Pete was treated with a nine-month course of Vivitrol. He's continued to visit restaurants and bars. And he's been with clients who favored large quantities of alcohol.

But Pete doesn't want to drink anymore, and he hasn't

since that day at the steakhouse when his old favorite just didn't do it for him.

Vivitrol; a solution that required a doctor's visit once a month and costs a fraction of everything he'd paid for as yet. Pete, who'd spent just about his entire life selling things, was sold. To understand how Vivitrol helps take away Pete's desire to drink, it is best to understand first the role the brain plays in craving "good" things.

When someone drinks alcohol or even thinks about drinking alcohol, it stimulates dopamine production and essentially triggers a high. A brain such as Pete's that has been damaged by alcohol takes these thoughts and turns them into an urge to drink, even if no alcohol is in sight. So, even though Pete might have been trying to stay sober, his brain could continue providing wrong messages. In essence, Pete's brain would get locked in a battle with itself. The logical reasons for alcohol abstention come from the cerebral cortex, the rational part of the brain, and face off against the limbic response system, the emotional center.

When Pete is exposed to a trigger, dopamine production begins automatically. The pleasant memories of his drinking surface and the craving begins.

The drug, Vivitrol, is meant to help dramatically cut down on cravings. Because of this, it is known as an "opioid antagonist." An antagonist is something that binds to a receptor in the brain and blocks its effects. In Pete's case, drinking targets opioid receptors, which then stimulate unusually high levels of dopamine production when he thinks about drinking or craves alcohol. That is also the same chain of events that occurs when he consumes alcohol.

An antagonist can act almost like gum in the ignition lock of a car. When gum gets stuck in the ignition lock, it makes it impossible for a key to start the car. Vivitrol is an opioid antagonist that fits into opiate receptors. In essence, it keeps the car from starting; it prevents the response of pleasure that is usually produced by drinking alcohol.

Vivitrol: Fighting the Urge to Relapse

To be most effective, treatment with Vivitrol, as the oral form of naltrexone, should begin after a person has completely withdrawn from alcohol. That means a person must avoid drinking for three to seven days before treatment begins. That may be achieved via a detox center or by spending time in an alcohol rehabilitation center.

There are schools of thought, mostly in 12-step recovery programs such as AA, that believe that in order to avoid relapsing into alcohol use disorder, a person must maintain complete abstinence from drinking. With counseling alone, however, statistics prove that 70 percent of alcoholics will relapse within one year. And, some say, up to 80 percent of alcoholics either can't or won't stop drinking.

Vivitrol is designed to take into consideration an individual with alcohol use disorder's tendency to relapse. The drug may help reduce the number of days a person drinks each month, as well as the number of drinks consumed. It helps people like Pete abstain from alcohol as part of their ongoing recovery.

For instance, when Pete is on Vivitrol and in a situation where alcohol is present, his brain may still wrestle with the belief that having one drink won't do any harm. But if Pete actually consumes an alcoholic drink, as he did when he was at the steakhouse, the opioid receptors don't generate the same "high" that he experienced before treatment. Vivitrol blocks the opioid receptors. Often, a person will put down the drink midway through, or finish one drink and not have anymore. This is what happened to Pete.

The COMBINE Study

Vivitrol, which is the injectable form of naltrexone, does not take the place of alcohol counseling. A combination of counseling and medicine often offers alcoholics their best chance of recovery. But the therapy need not be of the intense, daily variety that characterizes 12-step programs like AA.

The COMBINE (Combining Medications and Behavioral Interventions for Alcoholism) Study, which was published in 2006, confirmed the effectiveness of naltrexone. The study essentially demonstrated that long-term, intensive therapy might not be that helpful or necessary.

Of the COMBINE Study's nine treatment groups, the group that had brief counseling interventions paired with naltrexone had the most success for keeping alcoholics sober over the long haul. This group performed better than the next two top-scoring groups. Coming in second was a group that had brief medical counseling and intensive cognitive-behavioral therapy (CBT) but no naltrexone. In third was the group whose results were most surprising; that group received naltrexone, brief medical counseling, *and* intensive CBT. This group proved that more counseling does not necessarily translate into better results.

Overcoming Drug Adherence Issues

Using Vivitrol helps extend the effectiveness demonstrated by naltrexone in the COMBINE Study. Because Vivitrol is medically administered by physicians (in the buttocks), it takes away the issues of patient self-compliance that are associated with oral naltrexone. With the requirement of a daily pill, some alcoholics look at themselves in the bathroom mirror, pill in hand, as their brain wrestles with the idea of whether they really don't want to drink that day.

An injection of Vivitrol lasts 30 days (one month) and is designed to prevent the alcoholic's brain from wrestling with that daily decision. And for a person who is dependent on alcohol, part of that decision includes factoring in the role of deception. Many get caught up thinking they can "get away with drinking, today."

Having scheduled visits for Vivitrol injections mean that a spouse, other family members, or friends know where a person should be at a certain time each month - in the doctor's office. If the person doesn't show up for their shot, the naltrexone will have left their system. Within days, when they've potentially come home drunk, their secret is revealed, and that feeling of having let down their family comes flooding back.

With the shot, the question of "Do I want to take something that will prevent me from enjoying alcohol tonight?" becomes a moot point. And it stays moot for the month that the naltrexone remains in a person's system.

Vivitrol helps an alcoholic feel what life is like without the alcohol "high" for at least one month. If a person does drink alcohol, all the unpleasant effects of being drunk, like slurred speech and drowsiness, may be triggered, but none of the pleasant ones which alcoholics crave will return. This means, as with Pete, that the first drink a person may have is often their last.

Studies found that the drug was generally well-tolerated and produced mild to moderate side effects similar to oral naltrexone, the most prominent being nausea.

A course of the treatment can last three months to one year or longer. With several months of abstinence strung together, a person whose life used to revolve around alcohol has an ever-increasing chance of long-term abstinence. Thanks to Vivitrol, Pete was able to entertain clients, watch his beloved team win (or lose), be a reliable husband and father, and maintain sobriety.

Vivitrol essentially gives the brain a chance to reconfigure itself - separating good signals from bad ones and making more logical connections. The one side effect Pete experienced with Vivitrol was an injection-site reaction. That happened with a few other shots Pete had over the years, but the reaction usually cleared up quickly after taking a non-drowsy antihistamine. And the tradeoff of a little itching was certainly worth the complete difference the drug made in Pete's life.

For "the Answer Man," Vivitrol was finally his answer.

Review

What was happening to Pete?

Pete felt a lot of pressure at work and thought that younger associates were passing him over.

He speculated that the company was going to "show the old guy the door."

Pete's wife seemed to be slowing down and spending more time asleep, leaving him alone with his thoughts.

What was happening in Pete's brain?

When Pete was drinking alcohol, or even thinking about it, the production of the chemical, dopamine, was stimulated, essentially triggering a high.

Pete's brain, damaged by alcohol, interpreted false signals as an urge to drink even when no alcohol was in sight.

Although Pete was trying to stay sober, his brain continued to provide wrong messages and his craving for alcohol would kick in.

How did Pete get prescribed naltrexone/Vivitrol?

Pete was given a test called AUDIT (Alcohol Use Disorders Identification Test), developed by the World Health Organization to screen people for at-risk drinking and alcohol use disorder.

Pete's doctor had recently read the NIAAA publication Helping Patients Who Drink Too Much: A Clinician's Guide, and had also learned about the availability of alcohol recovery drugs that he could administer.

Why was Pete a good candidate for Vivitrol?

To be most effective, treatment with Vivitrol should begin after a person has completely withdrawn from alcohol. For most people, that means their withdrawal must have been completed at least 3 to 7 days beforehand, and Pete fits those criteria.

Vivitrol takes into consideration an individual with alcohol use disorder's tendency to relapse. The medicine may help reduce the number of days a person drinks each month as well as the number of drinks consumed.

Given Pete's exposure to alcohol on a regular basis during client meetings, Vivitrol was suggested because it can control alcohol cravings and nearly eliminate "slips" that can lead to full-blown relapses.

Pete's lifestyle fits well with having the Vivitrol administered via injection once per month by a medical professional.

What does naltrexone/Vivitrol do?

Naltrexone:

Gained approval from the FDA in 1994.

Works by reducing the desire for alcohol.

Interferes with parts of the brain that produce pleasure from drinking.

Vivitrol:

The injectable form of naltrexone administered once per month in the buttocks, can control alcohol cravings and nearly eliminate slips that can lead to major relapses.

May reduce cravings significantly.

Will not interfere with the parts of their brain responsible for all types of pleasure, just on the parts of the brain connected with the "alcohol high."

* * *

Signature Reflection: The Answer Man

Pete doesn't lose his life in one dramatic collapse - he loses it in small permissions: one more drink, one more deal, one more night where the body pays tomorrow for today. The story is a portrait of quiet decline - and quiet reversal, when treatment becomes specific and consistent.

If you remember one thing: recovery is built from repeated, ordinary choices.

- The dragon's disguise: charm, success, and "I can handle it."
- The turning point: an honest inventory, structured support, and medication that reduces reinforcement.
- A practice to try: name your highest-risk ritual and design a sober replacement before the next temptation.

Clinical lens: naltrexone blocks opioid-mediated reinforcement; long-acting injectable forms can reduce adherence barriers. The science works best when paired with a plan: follow-up, counseling, and relapse-prevention routines.

The Whizz Kid

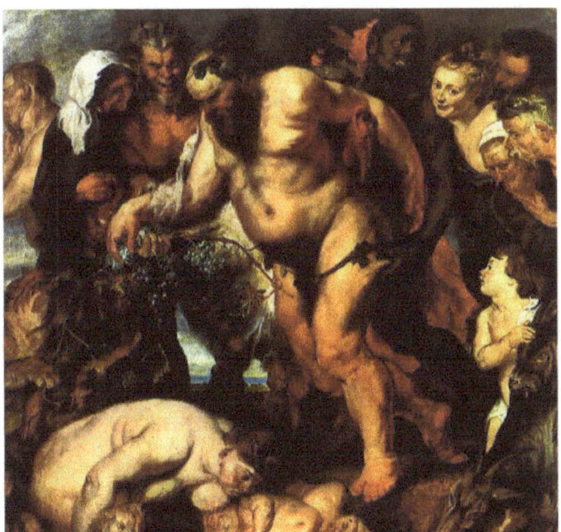

The image above is: Drunken Silenus - Peter Paul Rubens.

Peter Paul Rubens's *Drunken Silenus* holds myth and warning in the same frame: the tutor of Dionysus, said to grow cleverer as he drinks, carried by a crowd that celebrates him even as it steadies his staggering weight.

Rubens does not romanticize the cost. The body is swollen and heavy, reshaped by excess. It is a fitting doorway into Mark's story - a mind that runs like lightning, and a life that learns to use alcohol as both fuel and eraser, until medicine and accountability offer a different kind of rescue: not gold, but clarity.

Topiramate, the medication featured in this story, can help by quieting the excitatory drive that amplifies craving and by shifting the reward balance back toward choice. But the deeper work is still human: building a life where brilliance does not require anesthesia.

The Philadelphia web-development company had become a leader in building immersive sites for Fortune 500 clients. Eight years earlier it had started in a basement. Now it was scaling faster than anyone expected, because it was betting on the future - forums, games, video, tools that made a website feel like a world.

On the door to Mark's small, windowless office, the slogan had evolved. '2.0' was crossed out, replaced with '2.5,' then '3.0,' and finally '3.14159' - pi, the number that never ends. People joked that Mark's mind worked the same way: no finish line, just more possibility.

Mark came from comfort - his father a patent attorney, his mother a senior HR manager - but he never wore it like armor. He volunteered, tutored younger kids in math, and became senior class president because people trusted him.

He'd been building websites since he was fifteen, making enough on the side to buy new software, games...and beer.

This Philadelphia-based web development company had

become a leader in creating innovative websites for Fortune 500 companies, despite having had a humble beginning, taking off from its founder's basement barely eight years earlier. The company had seen the future in developing online forums, games, video, and other site-specific tools, and its vision was paying off.

On the door to Mark's small, windowless office at TruTech was that same sign...only, the figure '2.0' was crossed out; first to say '2.5,' then '3.0,' and, finally, '3.14159,' representing the mathematical term 'pi' that runs for an infinite number of decimal places. Those around him felt that Mark could have adopted the last name 'Pi' because there seemed to be no end to what he could do.

Despite an upbringing that some called privileged (Dad was a patent attorney, Mom, a senior human resources manager for an accounting firm), he never put on airs. He was considered generous to a fault, always among the first kids at school to volunteer for projects that varied from cleaning up the campus to helping tutor elementary school kids in math. His gregariousness eventually landed him the post of senior class president.

Mark had gained a reputation as a whiz kid. He'd been designing sites since he was 15, making enough money on the side to keep buying the latest software, games...and beer.

He always seemed to have a few bucks around to pay some adult to walk into the liquor store and buy a few six-packs. The beneficent adult would turn the beer over to Mark, who'd have strategically positioned himself in the parking lot beyond the watchful eye of store clerks. Each time Mark and his friends retreated to someone's basement, he cemented his reputation as the "Pied Piper of Ale." And when Mark and his friends met in the basement of his family's house, there was always the opportunity to taste his parents' supply of the hard stuff. Dad favored vodka; Mom liked gin.

Mark eventually entered an Ivy League college. As a freshman, he could hold his alcohol like only a few around him. On any given Friday or Saturday night (and sometimes Thursday nights), he could drink about six beers, the only effects being frequent bathroom visits. In the second semester of his freshman year, he became a natural fit for a fraternity.

He upheld his reputation as a whiz kid through his first two years at school. While becoming one of the more recognized figures on campus, he maintained a near 4.0 GPA and held a work-study job on the school's website. The job paid 15 hours' worth of wages for work that he usually completed in about 7 hours. He was active in his fraternity's service projects, tutoring kids from an adjoining neighborhood, raising money for heart disease research, and representing the frat at intra-campus meetings.

At the beginning of his junior year, Mark was elected treasurer of his fraternity. What better person to handle the finances of a group of 75 young men? And who better than a guy who'd been buying beer since he was 15 to figure out how the frat's alcohol budget could be stretched to the limit?

Even more incredible, the 10 beers he was drinking on Friday nights, Saturday nights, and sometimes Thursday nights and Sunday afternoons didn't seem to be affecting his GPA.

His First Incident

The finances of Mark's fraternity were thriving. He'd figured out ways to promote the frat's parties on the Web and have people willingly hand over $10 admission fees.

The frat's Halloween bash was on target to be the biggest blowout the school had ever seen. Mark had arranged to have a graveyard laid out on the front lawn, rented smoke machines, hired a local acting troupe to play flesh-eating zombies, and lined the house's interior with black lighting, hanging bats, cobwebs, and eerie-looking swamp trees. He hired bartenders to serve orange-colored beer and mixed drinks.

By most accounts, the bash was a success. There had been a few minor scuffles during the party, but each situation was diffused quickly. That was until about 2 a.m.

Mark, wearing a mummy costume, was working on his 15th beer of the night, and decided, out of the blue, that two cars parked in front of the house would make excellent trampolines. He convinced three other frat buddies that jumping on these cars would be a "great idea!" With nearly three hundred onlookers, Mark, dressed as an Egyptian mummy with requisite tattered white cloth strips, scaled the hood of a Honda Accord and began to bounce up and down like he was on springs.

He soon made his way to the vehicle's roof, where he began to dance a bizarre combination of an Irish jig, the Twist, and something from the Broadway production of "Guys and Dolls." His three frat buddies tried to keep up with his moves, but they mostly just jumped up and down.

"On three!" yelled Mark. "One..." The crowd joined in the count. "Two... Three!"

With that, Mark and his three friends vaulted from the trunk of the Accord onto the hood of a Jeep. The Jeep's roof had more room than the Accord's, and it accommodated the antics of four people simultaneously.

To the hoots and hollers of the crowd, the four frat brothers set the following sequence in motion:

JUMP

JUMP

JUMP

CRACK!

The "crack" was the sound of the Jeep's roof beginning to cave in.

One frat brother jumped off the car, then another, then another, leaving Mark as the lone "roof dancer."

JUMP! CRACK!

JUMP! CRACK!

JUMP! CRACK!

And then...there was the sound of sirens, followed by the sight of four campus security vehicles and six municipal police cars.

Within five minutes, in front of an astonished crowd, three municipal policemen were escorting someone out of the fraternity house and down its long driveway. Three men were dressed in blue law enforcement uniforms; the man they were escorting looked like he'd stepped out of the year 1000 B.C. with a trail of tattered white cloth strips. The officers helped the mummy into the back seat of a police car and formed a convoy with the other law enforcement vehicles to escort this "misplaced stranger" to jail.

Signature Scene: The Morning After

Mark woke to a mouth like sandpaper and a stomach that felt bruised from the inside. The mummy costume lay twisted on the floor like shed skin. His phone vibrated against the nightstand - too many notifications, too much light, too much proof that the night had kept going after his memory stopped.

He sat up slowly, letting the room settle. A dull ache pulsed behind his eyes. When he blinked, the images came back in broken flashes: the roof of the Jeep bending under his feet, the crowd's laughter turning sharp, the sound of a crack that didn't feel funny anymore. Then sirens - red and blue light slicing through smoke and music.

His laptop was open on the desk, screen dimmed but not asleep. Lines of code stared back at him like a language he'd suddenly forgotten. He tried to read, tried to think, and felt something he almost never felt: lag. The whiz kid part of him stuttered. The fear that rose was clean and new - *what if I've broken the one thing I'm good at?*

In the kitchenette down the hall, a half-empty case of beer sat under the counter from someone's weekend run. Mark's hand hovered over it without him deciding to move. He could already taste the relief. He could also taste the shame. He closed the cabinet hard enough to make the dishes rattle, then leaned on the sink, breathing like he'd just sprinted.

It wasn't that he didn't understand consequences. It was

that alcohol had started to erase the space where consequences were supposed to live. The night before, he had felt invincible. Now, with the sunlight pressing through the blinds, he understood the true risk: not that he drank, but that when he drank, he stopped steering.

The Aftermath

"Well...you've gotten yourself into quite a mess," said the college's dean of disciplinary affairs. "You're lucky we have a good relationship with the city police."

Following the Halloween bash, Mark had been charged with disorderly conduct, destroying property, public lewdness, and intent to serve alcohol to minors.

"You know the school has every right to ask you to leave," the dean said. "But you do have a record of being a good student and contributing to the welfare of the school. Between the school's insurance and the insurance held by the drivers of both vehicles that you seemed to enjoy treating like matchbox cars, the damage you caused will be covered."

"However..." the dean added, "the city and the university are asking that you complete a 90-day program at Alcoholics Anonymous. You are to attend meetings three times per week. After each meeting, you need to have the group leader sign forms certifying that you've attended. Once you complete the program to the satisfaction of both the city and the school, the charges against you will be dropped. Additionally, you're going to have to resign your post as fraternity treasurer."

To Mark, it sounded like a good deal. He could live without being treasurer. But he only thought of himself as a binge drinker - not an alcoholic. He wasn't drinking all the time. But if he had to attend AA to get out of this mess, he'd do it.

Being directed to AA by high schools and colleges is fairly common. These educational institutions often ask students who have been identified as having "problems with alcohol," not necessarily proven as "alcoholics," to attend AA meetings. People in their teens and 20s actually represent the fastest-growing segment of AA membership. And when Mark attended AA meetings, he became part of the sizable percentage of members who were forced to join, mostly by the healthcare and justice systems.

College-Age Drinking and its Consequences

The significant features of the American Psychiatric Association's definition of an alcohol use disorder, as put forth in its Diagnostic and Statistical Manual of Mental Disorders, Fifth Edition (DSM-5), are:

A preoccupation with drinking

Impaired control over drinking

Compulsive drinking

Drinking despite physical or psychological problems caused or made worse by drinking, alcohol tolerance, and/or withdrawal symptoms.

Alcohol use among emerging adults is quite common, and much of it can be categorized as "hazardous." For instance, binge drinking remains frequent among college students despite increased calls for its prevention. Up to 40 percent of college students have binged within the past two weeks.

About 25 percent of college students have had drinking-related academic problems such as missing classes, falling behind, doing poorly on exams and papers, or getting lower grades.

Binge drinking contributes to between 1,500 and 1,700 deaths - and 600,000 injuries (200,000 serious ones) - yearly amongst U.S. college-age students. It also increases health risks and psychosocial consequences, including incidences of:

Motor vehicle accidents

Legal problems

Personal injuries

Date rape

Violence

Depression

Unwanted or unprotected sex

Sexually transmitted diseases

Blackouts

In 2001 alone:

Nearly 700,000 students between ages 18 and 24 were assaulted by another college student who had been drinking.

More than 400,000 students had unprotected sex.

100,000 reported being too intoxicated to know whether or not they had consented to sex.

Alcohol use in emerging adults increases during such events as spring break, when low impulse control combines with higher rates of casual sex and reduced availability of condoms.

Serious drinking or binge drinking among college students can lead to long-term health problems, even among those who don't experience alcohol-related injuries. People who drink severely or binge drink between ages 18 and 24 are more likely to become alcohol dependent or alcohol abusers.

About 31 percent of college students meet the diagnostic criteria for alcohol abuse and 6 percent for alcohol dependence. Severe or binge drinking during college may predict the likelihood of having alcohol-related disorders up to 10 years later.

The average age when alcohol dependence (alcoholism) begins is 22, but the onset varies most often from the mid-teens to age 25, though there are some instances of onset that reach into middle age and later.

But in the 2001-2002 NIAAA study, called the National Epidemiologic Survey on Alcohol and Related Conditions (NESARC), alcoholism was found to be most prevalent among adults between ages 18 and 29.

Despite the identification of a mean age for the onset of alcohol dependence, research continues to find that alcoholism defies conventional perceptions.

Many heavy drinkers do not have alcohol dependence. Among people who have 5 or more drinks a day, the rate of alcohol dependence's development is less than 7 percent per year.

Most people who develop alcohol dependence have a mild-to-moderate disorder characterized primarily by impaired control. Such people may set drinking limits but exceed them or have trouble quitting or cutting down. Generally, these people do not experience severe alcohol-related problems with relationships, health, work, or the law.

Just 13 percent of people who are alcoholics receive specialty alcohol treatment.

Getting Back in the Swing of Things

By the end of his junior year's spring semester, Mark was back to his old drinking patterns. Having six beers a night on Thursdays through Sundays was consistent. He went as high as 10 on Fridays and Saturdays. He was no longer the treasurer of the fraternity, but he was still a brother. His GPA still flirted within the 4.0 mark, which suggested that the effects of the alcohol certainly weren't showing up in his academic performance. He was still at his work-study job and tutoring kids in Math when he had the chance.

As he entered his senior year, Mark felt like the world was his oyster. He knew so many people through his fraternity, his classes, and his work that he never needed to ask anyone if they wanted to go hang out at one of the campus bars. He always knew he'd eventually run into somebody.

By the end of September, with the fraternity capitalizing on his precedent of holding large parties, he found himself in a great position to meet women. Relieved of the day-to-day treasurer duties, he felt freer to "work the room." For some reason, his senior status seemed to be attracting women he thought would never have given him a second look.

While at his fraternity's Fall Festival party, he noticed that a beautiful woman was giving him the eye. He wasn't sure if he was seeing her through the haze of "beer goggles," although he did wonder whether the 10 beers he'd already consumed were making everyone seem good-looking.

He struck up a conversation with her, and the two became a little "touchy-feely." By beer 14, he decided to take her up to his room.

And that was all he could remember; he'd apparently

blacked out. His memory of what happened while he was with the woman from the party was utterly gone.

The next morning, he woke with a pounding headache. Nothing that he hadn't experienced before and nothing that a bunch of aspirin couldn't fix. He was all set to go to breakfast with a few fraternity brothers when he realized the $100 previously on his desk was missing. After one of his brothers agreed to pick up the tab on his meal, he began reconstructing some of the previous night's events.

"Dude," said one of his brothers, "I don't know what you were thinking. That girl was a major skank! I mean, she might have looked okay from where you were standing, but she was dressed like a 'ho' waiting for the Navy to pull into port."

No one at the table had recognized the woman Mark had been with. None of them had ever seen her, or the people she came with, on campus. Assuming he'd never see her again, Mark put the matter to rest.

About a month later, however, Mark began experiencing a burning sensation during urination. A visit to the student health service confirmed that he had contracted gonorrhea.

So Mark's night of 15 beers had resulted not only in his blacking out and having sex with a complete stranger, but also in the acquisition of a sexually transmitted disease because of his failure to use a condom.

Standard protocol is to treat the person infected with gonorrhea first and then ask that person to contact all the other people with whom he or she has had sexual contact. That way, everyone can be treated.

Mark had no way of contacting the woman he'd had sex with at the party, the one who must have given him the infection. But he was able to speak with the sophomore communications major he'd started seeing just three weeks earlier. He knew it was best to tell her and suggest she get evaluated, but there was no happy ending after the discussion. The woman told him flat out that this tale indicated she could not trust his judgment, especially when he could not identify the person who infected him.

This incident put Mark in a funk for one of the rare times in his life. Though he'd maintained good grades and a reputation for solid class attendance, he spent the first week of November skipping most of his classes. His usual routine of drinking anywhere from 6 to 10 beers on Friday and Saturday nights, along with some Thursday nights and Sunday afternoons, stretched into Sunday night.

When he felt like crap on Monday morning, Mark decided to sleep in until noon. When Monday night rolled around, one of the campus bars was having a special of 10-cent wings and $2 pitchers during the football game. He managed to grab a few fraternity brothers and snag a table about 10 feet from the big-screen TV that was showing the game.

On Tuesday, he decided to blow off his morning class but attended his 11 a.m. advanced Web design course. In the afternoon, before he was due to report to his work-study job, he called in sick.

On Tuesday night, his fraternity was showing DVD movies in the house's lounge area. Scheduled was one of the final *Star Trek* films to feature the original crew of the Starship Enterprise. Many in attendance turned movie night into a drinking game.

Every time the starship physician, Dr. McCoy, said, "Damn

it, Jim!" participants would have to take a swig of beer; every time engineer Scotty said, "I need more power!" participants would have to drink a shot of whiskey.

On Wednesday morning, Mark stayed in bed. He was determined to blow off all his classes for the day. Wednesday night was basically quiet, just five beers with dinner.

On Thursday, Mark thought he might be getting back on track. He hit his 8:30 class, followed by a 10:30 class and sometime in the library; at 2 p.m., he reported to his work-study job and finished what he needed to do by 6 p.m.

This led to Thursday evening, another drink-special night at campus bars. Mark was able to get pints of a British stout for just $2. Continuous servings of wings, cheese fries, and something else that was breaded and fried helped balance his beer intake. By the time he was ready to head home at about 1 am, his drinking tally had included four pints of stout, three imported ales, three American lagers, and three whiskey chasers.

On Friday morning, with his head pounding, Mark decided that the weekend had really begun the night before. He blew off all his classes and settled in for a long day of challenging friends to video games.

By the following Monday, after another weekend of drinking and parties, he got himself back to class and back on schedule.

In the second semester of his senior year, with the finish line of graduation in sight, Mark was attempting to carry six classes for a total of 18 credits. He exceeded his expected course load of five classes when he figured out that completing the extra class (Accounting 403) would give him a dual major in Engineering Digital Media Design as well as Business.

But as his semester progressed, he found himself attending Accounting 403 less and less. The scheduled class time of 8:30 a.m. on Monday, Wednesday, and Friday (especially Mondays) didn't really jibe well with his dedication to drinking. Time after time, he rationalized his absences by saying to himself, "Who wants to get up that early on Monday after a hard night of watching a Sunday night football game? I'll catch up on Wednesday."

By the end of his senior year, Mark's academic ambition waned. He decided to drop Accounting 403 because he'd missed so many classes. He would remain just three credits shy of a dual major. For all he'd miss about hanging with his fraternity brothers, graduation couldn't come quickly enough.

He knew he would be fine once he finished school. Job applications to Web development companies that he had sent at the urging of instructors were bringing interest. He would be able to make good money once he started, though he could expect some long hours. Maybe he would combine beer and energy drinks to keep going.

The "Urban Fringe" Drinker

The population that sociologists call "Cyber Millennials" [sic], tech-savvy singles and couples living in urban fringe neighborhoods, has the highest rate of risky drinking in the U.S. "Urban fringe" refers to more affordable, up-and-coming neighborhoods just outside of more established areas.

This segment of the young adult generation is often well educated, ethnically mixed, and technologically sophisticated. They tend to be among the most health-conscious segments of society, with lower smoking rates and vows to work out and eat organic produce. Yet their binge drinking tendencies clearly go against their basic commitment to healthy lifestyles.

These young, seemingly healthy patients tend not to raise questions among physicians. Many doctors don't even ask about a "Cyber Millennial's" [sic] level of alcohol consumption or provide screens for alcohol problems. Yet, up to half of all high-risk drinkers are young adults.

Three Years Later

Having spent time in the employ of TruTech, and making good money (more than many of his peers from high school and college were taking in), Mark took his dad's advice and decided to buy a condo. Embracing the mantra of "location, location, location," he set his sights on up-and-coming areas of Philadelphia, not far from his Center City office. His realtor called these areas "fringe" neighborhoods - places that feel a little like an "urban village."

He decided to make his purchase in the Northern Liberties neighborhood, barely 1.2 miles from the Liberty Bell. He could walk to work on some days and take a bus or train on others.

The neighborhood was beginning to experience growth with new businesses and restaurants. But what hit him the most was the fact that his new condo was down the block from Doc's, a place with an art-deco feel that was half bowling alley, half retro-lounge, and all the rage among people in his age group. When looking at homes, he saw a sign near Doc's front door that listed the Wednesday special:

After 10 p.m.
$2 shoes, $2 bowling, $2 tater tots,
$2 American and Mexican beers

Mark made Doc's *his* place on most Wednesdays. Things worked out well on those days. He could work until about 9:30 p.m., drop off his laptop at home, and get to Doc's just in time for the special to begin. He was respected enough in the office to be allowed to start work at 10:30 a.m. on Thursdays, so staying out late wasn't an issue.

He'd gotten to know a few people in his building who also favored Doc's on Wednesdays, so hanging out there felt a little like college. Though he was three years out of school, his drinking patterns hadn't changed much. He'd shifted one of his drinking nights to Wednesday instead of Thursday, but Friday and Saturday nights, as well as Sunday afternoons, were usually filled with suds.

As busy as his life seemed to be, consisting mostly of a "work hard, play hard" mentality, Mark found time to have a girlfriend. The lovely Sydney, who'd moved to Philly from Pittsburgh to join a mid-sized law firm, became the person with whom he spent the most time. Given her work schedule, she respected the commitment Mark had made to his employer. Mark never felt smothered by her, and that was part of her charm.

As he gained seniority at his Web design firm, Mark found himself working on some of its biggest accounts. He designed games for the website of a major bank that was meant to teach kids how to save money. He created a graphic interface for a major sneaker manufacturer that would allow people to "build" their own shoe, from the thread style to the thread color. And his personal favorite was implementing tools for a beer company that would allow users to follow the journey of wheat and hops through the brewing process all the way to their lips.

But each big client brought the prospect of more deadlines. Mark enjoyed the chance to be creative and come up with solutions, and the major players at his company thought of him as a big piece of the puzzle. But with so much pressure, he found that he needed more frequent releases.

Doc's had some good specials during Monday night football games, and Mark found that the place was just as good on Mondays as it was on Wednesdays. For $20 he could have six beers and a plate of nachos, and still have money left over for tips.

On Thursdays, when he got home from work around 8 p.m., he could always turn to his fridge for a cold six-pack. That would usually be enough to vault him into the weekend barely 24 hours later.

But Fridays were now starting to feel like Mondays back at school when he signed up for Accounting 403 and found it unbearable to be up at 8:30 a.m. At least three times over the course of two months, he called in sick on a Friday.

And Mondays weren't feeling too good either. He called in sick on three separate Mondays over that same period of time.

Things were changing for Mark. Work was beginning to annoy him. The lovely Sydney was "on his case" about a decision to avoid driving to Pittsburgh to meet her parents. And the price of tater tots at Doc's had just jumped to $3.

His productivity at work was slowing. When he called in sick on a Friday and again on Monday - effectively giving him a four-day weekend - the Web design firm's V.P., John Standish, decided it was time to talk.

"Mark," said Standish, "You know we've always liked your work around here. You've been huge for us when it comes to some of our biggest accounts. But a few of us around here have noticed that you seem off your game over these last two or three months. You're calling in sick; you've been showing up in jeans and T-shirts.... I'm all in favor of personal expression, but sometimes that stuff has its limits, especially when it comes to your hair sticking straight up like you'd just stuck your finger in an electric socket.

"The hard truth is that we're in the business of making money here," the V.P. continued. "I want to give you as much leeway as possible, but you know how things work. We have a lot of clients who want things yesterday. And when you're not giving 100 percent, there are some deadlines we just can't meet. So tell me, what's going on?"

Mark scratched his head. He'd always been so good at what he did that this may have been the first time that he'd been told he wasn't living up to his end of the bargain. But Standish was one of the people who'd recruited him out of college, and he'd always had lots of respect for the man. He figured he could be upfront with him.

"Well," Mark said, "I'm not really sure. I've been putting in a lot of hours lately and my girlfriend, well...we've been fighting a bit. I think I might just be a little tired."

"I can respect that," said Standish. "It happens to the best of us. But I need to figure out a way to get you on your game. Look, how about this. Once you meet the deadlines on that carmaker account in two weeks, how about if you take two weeks off? Get your head together. Then, come back refreshed. Whaddaya say?"

"Uh...sounds good to me," said Mark.

Mark was buoyed by the idea of taking some time off. So much so that he skipped his Wednesday "appointment" at Doc's and started looking at last-minute travel sites.

During the two weeks that Mark would be off, Sydney would only be able to get away for three business days. So Mark booked a five-day Bahamas cruise out of Fort Lauderdale running Wednesday through Sunday. He figured they could fly down late Tuesday during his second week off, board the ship on Wednesday and fly back to Philly late on Sunday. He found out that he could stay for the rest of the time at a fraternity brother's house at the Jersey Shore.

Life's a Beach

When the time finally came to take his break, Mark threw whatever he needed into the back of his car and was down the shore in just over an hour. By the time he'd reached the shore house, the beer was already cold, and faces from his past mobbed him.

It didn't matter that he'd arrived at nearly 11 p.m.; there was still time to have "a few" beers. Mark managed to drink eight of them before 2:30 a.m.

When the sun finally nudged him awake on Saturday, he felt like he didn't have a care in the world. He had resolved to have a beer for breakfast, lunch, and dinner. Between meals, he would have beer on the beach, and his nights would be filled with his usual methods of consumption. By the time the day was done at about 3 a.m., Mark had begun to count the number of beers he'd had, using his fingers and toes.

"Let's see," Mark recounted. "There was the beer at breakfast, the two I had on the beach before lunch, the two I had at lunch, the four I had while on the beach in the afternoon, two at dinner and ten more after we went out. That's...twenty-one beers! I think that might be my new record!"

Sunday was much the same, though by Sunday night, he'd switched over to light beer. At least it was less filling.

On Monday, when crowds at the Jersey Shore eased due to work schedules, he found himself whiling away the hours playing "drinking Scrabble" with a few friends. In each round, the person with the lowest word score had to drink half a beer. Mark considered himself an excellent Scrabble player, but when friends asserted that words he'd constructed, including "metabolination" and "sarcocineous," were not actually words, he found himself on the short end of the stick. But that didn't bother him too much.

Tuesday's adventures were marked by a trip to a local bar called McMillan's Big Net. Not thinking about his upcoming cruise with Sydney, he decided to do a little flirting. He and his friends made conversation with a group of women who seemed nice enough. Mark began talking with a blonde. He had trouble identifying whether she was more like a sea captain or stockbroker and couldn't remember having ever spent time with a woman whose language was so salty. Still, he reasoned that he was at least having fun.

When he woke up Wednesday morning, he wasn't sure where he was. But there, lying next to him, was the woman his friends had dubbed "The Salty Dog."

He got up, felt the pockets of his jeans. In one of them was a single condom. That was actually good news, because he had taken two with him when the boys went out to McMillan's, and it probably meant that he'd remembered to use one during sex.

Mark's routine at the beach remained much the same through the remainder of his time there. Drink, eat, drink, eat, drink, eat...drink, drink, drink. He packed up his things late Tuesday morning of his second week away and drove back to Philly to prepare for his flight to Fort Lauderdale with Sydney. Going without beer for much of Tuesday would give him a chance to sober up, pack for the trip, and make it to the airport on time.

While waiting for his 7:30 p.m. flight, Mark grabbed a beer from a bar in the terminal. While in flight, he was able to buy two more. By the time he and Sydney reached their Fort Lauderdale hotel, it was already almost 11. Although he was ready for another drink, Sydney convinced him that since they needed to be on the ship by 9 a.m., getting some sleep wouldn't be such a bad idea.

When he woke up that Wednesday morning at 7 a.m., Mark found that he had a splitting headache. In the last 30 hours, he'd had only three beers; it was usually the other way around; he was used to taking a few aspirins after a night of hard-drinking, not after a night of almost *no* drinking.

"Is this what withdrawal feels like?" he thought.

For as beautiful as the cruise ship and the Bahamas were, the time he spent with Sydney seemed like the lowest point in their relationship. In the end, though, he was to blame.

There was the incident where he'd rented a wave runner and taken Sydney for a ride. Mark started to feel his oats and began jumping the waves made by a passing boat. Sydney pleaded with him to stop, but after their final jump, and after they'd fallen off the vehicle, the wave runner wouldn't start. They needed to catch a lift from the very same boat whose waves they'd flown over just minutes before.

All Mark could think was, "Man, I'm so glad this isn't the U.S. A breathalyzer test would probably be my worst enemy right now."

Then there was the incident after the midnight buffet. Mark, working on a plate of shrimp after having his 10th beer of the night, needed to rush out on deck to throw up. He almost made it to the ship's rail, but half of his vomit ended up on deck. Sydney ran out to attend to him, as a group of people in deck chairs tried not to stare.

And then, there was the "urine incident."

After a long day and night of drinking, Mark and Sydney returned to their cabin. Mark got up a number of times in the middle of the night to urinate; not once did his stream reach the toilet. When Sydney awoke to use the bathroom, she wanted to keep things dark so as not to wake Mark. When she walked there in her bare feet, she heard a low splash. When she finally turned on the light, she found her feet awash in a sea of urine.

Disgusted, she returned to bed and gave Mark the shove of a lifetime, watching him land on the floor with a heavy thud. Mark, not having the strength to get back in bed, spent the rest of the night sleeping on the floor.

Between the times they disembarked from the boat in Fort Lauderdale and exited the plane in Philadelphia, Sydney barely said a word to Mark. When he pulled up in front of her apartment to drop her off on Sunday night, she finally let him have it.

"What the hell is wrong with you!" she screamed. "I wanted to be with you because you were a nice guy - outgoing, friendly, and fun to talk to. You seemed to truly enjoy your neighborhood, the work you were doing, and the people you met along the way. I always knew you were partial to beer, but it never seemed to get in the way of the way you lived your life. That's just not true anymore.

"Now, you're a drunken bastard!" Sydney continued. "You drink constantly, you always have to make sure there's a beer within reach, and you're taking chances with your life...and mine! God knows what the hell you did when you were down the shore with your frat boy buddies!

"I think you're an alcoholic," Sydney finished. "And I think you need help."

"I'm not an alcoholic!" Mark shouted. "I like to drink beer. It's a part of my DNA! I can handle myself, I always have!"

"Look, until you get your life together, I don't want to see you," she said. "In fact, even if you sober up and get things straight, I'm not sure I'll ever want to see you. If we ever got married, what would I tell our kids? 'Daddy's a great guy except when he pees all over the floor and can't find his way home'? Yeah, that'll fly. Look, I'm no saint; I drink my share of beer too, but nothing like this!

"You're not in college anymore!" Sydney screamed. "Get things straightened out, or you're gonna end up dead! And do it soon! Goodbye, Mark."

And with that, she strode into her building, suitcase trailing behind, and never looked back.

I'm Fine

That first day back at work was tough for Mark. He looked neater, wearing a collared shirt and blue khakis, but his face looked a little too pale for someone who had spent two weeks in the sun. His eyes had dark circles, and he had stubble on his face that indicated he was toying with the idea of growing a goatee but had started much too late in the vacation.

He could feel his brain pulsating when he tried coming up with ideas for some new projects. He was going to need some aspirin even before he started drinking, which he was planning to do at Doc's later. Maybe it would help drown the sadness he felt over losing Sydney.

And so, he sank back into his routine. Drinking almost every night of the week, averaging between 6 and 15 beers; eating tater tots.

After about a month, he began calling in sick every other Friday. Then it became Friday and Monday. It wasn't long before Standish decided that he'd seen enough.

"Mark," he said. "It's fairly obvious to everyone here that you've got a problem. Whether its drugs, alcohol or whatever, it's not my concern. What is my concern is that you're falling behind in everything you do here, and as it stands now, I don't see any sign of you turning things around!"

Mark's heart sank. Again, he thought, "It can't be that bad...I am *NOT* an alcoholic!"

"Look, here's what I think you need to do," Standish said. "Go see Judy in HR, tell her you need to get familiar with the company's Employee Assistance Program (EAP). The EAP can probably set you up with some counseling and help you figure out what your next move is.

"This is something I think you've got to do," Standish went on. "You're just not the same ambitious, fun-loving guy we hired out of school. I know life gets more complicated as time goes on, but I have a feeling whatever you're doing is making things much harder. I want to see that old guy again. We need you around here. Go get fixed up, and let's get you back in the saddle. OK?"

Sobering Up

The company's EAP program helped Mark pick out a rehab facility. His insurance would cover seven to 10 days' worth of medically assisted withdrawal and 10 days of residential counseling. Most of the programs ran between 21 and 28 days, so if he wanted to complete them, Mark realized he'd have to pay the balance himself.

"Well, I won't be spending money on beer much anymore, so that's a start," Mark told himself.

He checked into a facility named The Peaceful Ranch near Lancaster, PA. The place was beautiful; fields and gentle, rolling hills surrounding it. He was able to watch Amish people drive by in their horses and buggies.

After eight days, he emerged from withdrawal feeling different from how he'd felt in years. At age 26, it was probably the longest he'd gone without alcohol since he was about 17. Things seemed clearer, and he no longer had that bloated feeling.

As his residential treatment began, he had a flashback to the 90 days he spent with AA. The center was dedicated to helping people sober up for the long haul by embracing AA's principles. The stories were just as wild. The invocation of help from a higher power was a little less fervent, but its presence was still ominous. He knew he could stick it out. It would give him ample opportunity to write a long, apologetic letter to Sydney, and at least it would give him about 30 days of sobriety to build upon.

Just prior to his discharge from The Peaceful Ranch, he was told that his name would be given to a few AA groups near his home and office. That way, he could work at his sobriety on a daily basis with people who'd "really been there."

The thought of having to go to AA - for essentially the rest of his life - was something that Mark couldn't bear to think of. Having seen how things worked for 90 days back in college was almost enough to make him want to jump off a bridge. Before leaving, he asked the Peaceful Ranch counselors whether they knew of any medicines that might help with his sobriety. Their answers included:

"There's no way to keep sober other than having faith in a higher power."

"Oh, they're out there, but they're expensive, and they don't work so well."

"You're an alcoholic, and you're gonna be an alcoholic for life! Taking drugs to get sober is like substituting crack for beer."

But Mark remembered reading that heroin addicts were given methadone to help them stay sober. Couldn't there be something that could help alcoholics stay sober?

Back Home

Upon his return to Philly, Mark remembered the name of a fraternity brother who was a few years older. Mark had heard that he was opening a family practice across the river in New

Jersey. So while he took the names of AA group leaders when he left The Peaceful Ranch, he figured that he would try to talk with a doctor first before subjecting himself to the torture of sobriety surrounded by stories of misery and religious enlightenment.

Dr. Gabe Cohen was about a year into his new practice in Cherry Hill. He had two partners, and the practice was gaining more patients by the month.

"So Gabe," Mark said, "You know I just did a stint in rehab to sober up from drinking."

"Wow," said Gabe. "That's a great thing. Congrats, man. I do remember that when you were pledging you certainly seemed like a guy who could throw back a few."

"Well, I don't want to go to AA," Mark continued. "I had to attend meetings for 90 days during college after that little incident. And it just never sat well with me. I need to find another way to keep sober before I fall off the wagon again. I feel good after drying out, but to tell you the truth, I still think about beer a lot."

"So let me ask you this," the doctor started. "For all these years you've been going to the doctor's, has anyone ever asked you about whether you ever used alcohol to excess?"

"Not one," Mark responded.

"Alright," said Gabe. "Hang here for a bit. Let me have you fill out these papers that detail you and your family's medical history. I'm going to get a few things so that we can give you a thorough physical."

When he returned, Gabe placed a stethoscope to Mark's chest.

"Ever hear of a drug called topiramate?" Gabe asked.

Mark: A Good Candidate for Topiramate

After Mark had filled out a personal and family health history, Gabe noticed that both of Mark's parents were heavy drinkers, though not necessarily alcoholics. He also noticed that Mark had a long and sustained history of very heavy drinking and that if he did not have a period of sustained low-level drinking, even if abstinence could not be attained immediately, his health would continue to spiral out of control.

Given that Mark presented with a sustained history of alcohol use disorder and that the immediate treatment goal was harm reduction, Dr. Cohen prescribed the drug topiramate.

Dr. Cohen had arrived at the idea of using topiramate to treat alcohol use disorder after reading the pioneering work of Professor Dr. Bankole Johnson, who invented this strategy and is the author of this book.

Topiramate is also sold under the brand name of Topamax. Originally approved for the treatment of epilepsy, topiramate is derived from a simple form of sugar known as monosaccharide D-fructose. It has the Food and Drug Administration (FDA) approval for preventing . Psychiatrists have used it to treat bipolar disorder and counteract the weight gain associated with some antidepressants. It has also been investigated for use in treating obesity, binge eating, posttraumatic stress disorder, bulimia, obsessive-compulsive disorder, smoking cessation, and cocaine dependence. It has not been approved by the FDA for treating alcoholism, but the experimental studies that have been published were very promising.

Topiramate appears particularly effective for reducing

cravings and increasing abstinence in people who are still drinking. Basically, there is no need for an alcoholic to become abstinent before taking topiramate - it can be given to them while they are still drinking heavily and finding it hard to stop. Indeed, Prof. Dr. Bankole Johnson's work had shown that a huge advantage of topiramate over any other medication was that the individual with alcohol use disorder could take it exactly when they needed it - when he or she was still drinking heavily!

Alcoholics receive pleasure from alcohol when it helps release the chemical dopamine in the brain. Topiramate essentially washes away excess dopamine and denies pleasure from drinking. First, it blocks the ability of the neurotransmitter, glutamate, to excite dopamine. Since glutamate is involved in the process of long-term memory, blocking it is like building a dam that holds back the pleasurable feelings associated with memories of drinking. Second, topiramate enhances the production of GABA. GABA accounts for alcohol's sedating effect on many brain functions, including judgment, movement, and breathing. The presence of more GABA means less dopamine output and, therefore, a reduction in the pleasurable effects of alcohol.

Topiramate enhances early and long-term abstinence. It further stabilizes moods and anxiety. It also was proven to be most effective when paired with brief counseling, such as BBCET (Brief Behavioral Compliance Enhancement Treatment) on a weekly basis. BBCET also was invented by the author in his search for a psychological way to help individuals in their family practitioner's clinic rather than at a self-help group.

BBCET can be as short as a weekly 15-minute session with a trained medical professional. Being able to get a medication that can work, and having one's own doctor provide the brief counseling, has the advantage of convenience (especially for alcoholics who are working or at school), privacy (no one else needs to know except you and your doctor), confidence that the regular meetings with the doctor will ensure that the course of the illness is followed closely, and - because the time commitment is small and rehab is not needed - greater contact with “real-life”, healthy and supportive relationships. In contrast, AA sessions vary greatly in length, often lasting more than an hour, and members are expected to attend several meetings a week, over the course of their lifetime.

Dr. Cohen had read that in two large-scale clinical trials, topiramate helped improve all drinking outcomes. One of the studies reported that heavy drinkers were six times more likely to remain abstinent for a month when taking topiramate even in small doses. Overall, the group taking topiramate ingested fewer drinks during a “drinking day,” had fewer heavy drinking days, had more days abstinent, and were less likely to binge drink when compared with the placebo group.

And half of everyone in the topiramate group reported less craving for alcohol; only 15 percent reported less craving in the placebo group.

In contrast, after three months of treatment, just two out of the 48 people in the placebo group (4 percent) were sober for, at least, one month.

Topiramate makes its way through the body, mostly unchanged before being excreted through urine. If Mark had experienced any liver impairment, the drug would not contribute to the worsening of any condition. Long-term studies have shown no serious problems related to the drug.

Treatment with topiramate usually begins with a dose of 25 mg/day. The dosage can be adjusted over a period of eight weeks to between 100 mg/day and 300 mg/day. It needs to be titrated slowly to avoid troublesome side-effects, and it is best to follow Prof. Dr. Bankole Johnson's first reported dosing sequence, which takes 8 weeks to reach the maximum dose. Most patients might, however, need to be treated for six months to one year to decrease the possibility of full-blown alcohol relapse. Topiramate can have side effects that include weight loss, fatigue, a feeling of pins and needles, mental slowness, and kidney stones. Topiramate may not be for everyone, but in all cases, the doctor has to balance the risks versus the rewards.

Importantly, the selection of topiramate for Mark was based on factors that were personalized towards him: high levels of binge drinking, a family history of an alcohol use disorder, difficulty achieving sobriety, and a focus on harm reduction.

Despite not being formally approved for the treatment of alcohol use disorder by the FDA, there has been so much reported success with topiramate that it has entered important national treatment guidelines such as the American Psychiatric Association Practice Guidelines for the pharmacological treatment of patients with alcohol use disorder.

Recently, there has been evidence that the effect of topiramate on glutamate receptors are most potent and selective for those that contain the GluK1 subunit (encoded by the gene glutamate receptor, ionotropic, kainate 1 [GRIK1]). If these findings are replicated, this will point to an even higher level of personalization in the use of topiramate for the treatment of alcohol use disorder.

Post-Treatment Success

Mark responded well to treatment with topiramate. Taking the drug strengthened the resolve he'd gained after rehab. In the first month, he was still tempted to drink, but early in month two, his desire was under control.

He missed hanging at Doc's. But not going there helped him realize how much of his time and energy had been devoted to drinking. His outgoing personality made it easy for him to meet people in his building who didn't drink so much, and he began following those people to the local gym. Time on a barstool was converted to time on a treadmill. Eventually, he joined a bicycling club. He even found a little time to tutor school-kids on Saturdays.

And fortunately for Mark, TruTech welcomed him back, this time as a stronger person who dressed neatly and showed up for work consistently. The sign reading *Welcome to Web 3.14159* was still on his door. Work felt easy again. He still wished the hours weren't quite as long, but he was regaining the satisfaction of being challenged.

Mark was enjoying his sobriety. And it occurred to him that Sydney had said she wouldn't even think about talking to him until he got his life in order. It had been eight months since he'd dropped her off at her front door. He'd sent her a long letter while in rehab but never heard anything back. Curiosity got the best of him, and he decided to send her a long e-mail telling her what he'd been up to.

The next day his cell phone rang. It was Sydney.

Review

Young Adults and Drinking

Half of all high-risk drinkers are young adults.

The population that sociologists call "Cyber Millennials" [sic], tech-savvy singles and couples living in urban fringe neighborhoods, has the highest rate of risky drinking.

Younger, healthier patients tend not to raise questions about alcohol use among physicians.

What Made Mark a Good Candidate for Topiramate

Mark filled out a family medical history for his doctor and received a thorough physical exam.

Both of Mark's parents were heavy drinkers.

He had a long and sustained history of very heavy drinking.

Without a long period of abstinence or even reducing his drinking to low levels, his doctor assessed that Mark's general health would continue to decline.

Mark became a good candidate because his doctor focused on an immediate treatment goal of harm reduction.

Harm reduction is a treatment that focuses on reducing the harm to a person's health caused by too much alcohol, with the goal of reducing alcohol intake first, rather than immediate abstinence.

Why Topiramate?

Topiramate has been proven effective in reducing cravings and increasing abstinence in people who are still drinking.

An alcoholic need not become abstinent before taking topiramate.

It works by essentially washing away excess dopamine and denying pleasure from drinking.

It enhances early and long-term abstinence and stabilizes moods and anxiety.

It was proven to be most effective when paired with brief counseling, such as weekly BBCET (brief behavioral compliance enhancement treatment).

BBCET can be as short as a weekly 15-minute talk with a trained medical professional, including a family doctor.

If Mark had experienced any liver impairment due to his long-term heavy drinking, the drug would not contribute to any worsening of the condition.

Most alcoholics need treatment with topiramate for six months to one year, to decrease the possibility of full-blown relapse.

* * *

Signature Reflection: The Whizz Kid

Mark's intelligence isn't the problem; it's the amplifier. The same speed that builds a career can also build a shortcut to numbness. This story offers a different hero arc: not genius, but steady repair - medicine, accountability, and a life designed for clarity.

If you remember one thing: your gifts need protection.

- The dragon's disguise: being "too capable" to need help.

- The turning point: accepting treatment and letting the brain de-escalate instead of constantly spiking.
- A practice to try: remove one automatic cue (a bar stop, a liquor aisle, a drinking app group chat) and replace it with a new cue.

Clinical lens: medications like topiramate can reduce craving by influencing excitatory-inhibitory balance. Pairing medication with brief, consistent counseling improves adherence and outcomes.

The Frequent Flyer

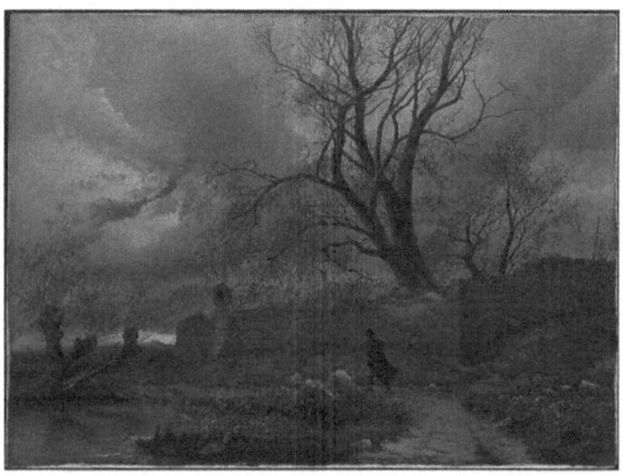

The image above is: Wanderer in the Storm (1835) - Julius von Leypold.

Julius von Leypold's *Wanderer in the Storm* (1835) holds a solitary figure against wind and weather - movement without shelter, progress without comfort. It echoes the spirit of Schubert's song cycle *Die Winterreise* (*Winter Journey*, 1827): travel as both escape and sentence.

In this story, the storm becomes flight - constant acceleration, constant distance. The leafless trees mirror

Maximillian's emotional barrenness. And the faint clearing on the horizon points to what he has not yet learned to believe in: that a targeted treatment plan, and the right clinician, can interrupt the trajectory before it turns fatal.

This public-domain work can also be viewed at the Metropolitan Museum of Art in New York.

Ultra-low-dose ondansetron, the medication featured here, reflects a hard truth and a hopeful one: the more precisely we understand the brain, the more precisely we can treat it. When Dragons Kill, they do not always roar. Sometimes they whisper, "You're fine - just keep moving."

At twenty-six he was the top trader at a mid-sized London securities firm. By thirty he was vice president. By thirty-five he was a regional VP at one of the world's largest brokerage houses. And by forty he had launched his own firm - SecureValue - flying between London and New York roughly fifteen times a year.

In a high-pressure industry that rewards certainty, very few people told Maximillian no. They didn't need to. He made money, and money made him untouchable - at least on paper.

When he walked into HR Owen's Rolls Royce dealership on the Old Brompton Road, no one said, "You're too young for this."

Maximillian had always lived in motion.

At age 26, he had become the top trader at a mid-sized London securities firm. By age 30, he was vice president of the firm. When he reached 35, he'd moved on to become a regional V.P. with one of the world's largest brokerage houses. And by 40, he'd started his own securities firm, SecureValue, whose operations kept him flying between London and New York about fifteen times per year.

During his rise to the top of a high-pressure, high-profile industry, very few people said 'no' to Maximillian. They didn't have to. He made his firm money and was rewarded highly for it. And making his clients money, won him constant praise.

When he showed up at HR Owen's Rolls Royce dealership on the Old Brompton Road in South Kensington, no one said, "You're too young to own one of these."

When he bought a mews house in Chelsea and then bought the one next door so he could knock down walls between the two and create an even bigger residence, no one said, "Don't do that." They only saw someone who had the means to keep the building "in fashion."

And when he threw holiday parties for the employees of his securities firm, nobody declined the invitation. That's because Maximillian had managed to do well for himself and those around him...despite his reputation as a lush.

His employees had come to admire him as a generous man who never failed to ensure their year-end bonuses. Though he had no children of his own, he always took time to ask about his employees' kids, and freely distributed tickets to Chelsea football club games around the company. Employees saw him as one of their own; a man who had grown up middle class and never put on airs, he gained their respect as a "character" for whom they enjoyed working.

Everyone knew it was bad form to spurn holiday party offers from the boss, even though most realized it would mean spending three hours watching Maximillian consume untold quantities of single-malt whiskey and transform from a pleasant host to a stumbling lunatic.

It wasn't like he hadn't tried to stop drinking. Maximillian had "stopped" plenty of times. But after a week, he'd usually end up plastered on the couch, watching reruns of classic Premier League games on Sky Sports 1.

"You could go on all you want," Maximillian used to say to anyone who would listen. "But no one ever played midfield better than Fàbregas. Fàbregas was *the* best! When you needed a pass at just the right time or a header that found its way through a crowd, Fabregas the marvelous was the man. Never be another like 'im."

He'd also attended AA meetings at the urging of a few friends. He was never particularly fond of the meetings but had made it so far at some points even to pick up a "sponsor." He tried keeping up with his sponsor, even when he felt the urge to drink on trips to New York, but his jet-setting lifestyle never made it easy to stick with AA and its philosophy of constant meetings, check-ins, and reminders to read the organization's *The Big Book* for guidance.

Rehab, Rehab, Rehab

As for rehab stints, Maximillian had done six of them. On his first three visits, his assistant, Margaret, set him up at a small facility in Wiltshire named Triumph. The place was more like a retreat - rolling hills, indoor and outdoor swimming pools, hiking trails, and massages - all at what seemed like the bargain price of £30,000/month.

Each time Maximillian left Triumph, he felt like a new man. A month clean and sober always had that effect on him. Yet each time, within four months of his release, he found himself back in the rolling hills of Wiltshire.

A bender of epic proportions preceded rehab stint number four. Maximillian spent weeks visiting pubs and treating the house to rounds of whiskey. As a chatty, outgoing fellow, he was never at a loss for conversation, and his ways ensured that he'd have long chats with 1, 2, or 75 people.

After that, he entered rehab at Hartsfield House in Kent. The place was purely pastoral. More like a farmhouse and petting zoo than say, a haven for drunks, pushers, and pill-poppers. A posh facility, yes, but Maximillian also learned how to milk a cow! Imagine all the conversations he could start with that one when talking to the boys from the trading floor. And at *only* £56,000/month!

Maximillian had managed to stay sober for six months after his first stint at Hartsfield House. But it all came crashing down after an elaborate argument at the Moon Dog pub in Clapham over who was a better goaltender, Peter Schmeichel or Gary Bailey.

"You're barmy!" Maximillian yelled. "I don't know how Bailey lasted so long! He made routine saves seem spectacular, but he couldn't cross to save his life. They didn't call him 'Dracula' for nothing. You're just talking bollocks!"

A crowd of 20 spilled into the street during that argument. Two Bobbies arrested Maximillian and six others and hauled them off to jail. After Maximillian was identified as being the instigator of the ruckus and he agreed to reimburse the owner for damages to the pub, he and the six others were allowed to go.

Back to Hartsfield. Another leisurely stay filled with milking cows and having counselors help him figure out just who he really was.

Six months later, while at a benefit dinner for Marie Curie Cancer Care, he didn't remember who he was. The organization's CFO was addressing the crowd with highlights of its past fundraising season. For some reason, Maximillian thought the man looked a lot like a sheepdog dressed in a tuxedo.

"And in June, we had our successful 10K run through Hyde Park," the CFO announced. "We had 10,000 participants and-"

"WOOF!"

It was Maximillian, from a table halfway between the stage and ballroom entrance.

"More important than the funds we raised, however, was the awareness that it helped to bring-"

"WOOF, WOOF!!!" called out Maximillian.

"Greater awareness to..." the CFO attempted to continue.

"Do you want a bone, Winston old boy?" called out Maximillian. "Here, ya go. FETCH!"

With that, Maximillian threw the steak bone from his plate at the stage. Hotel security then escorted him from the hall. As he was led away, he yelled out, "What? If you don't like bones, just say so! I can get you some biscuits in a flash!"

Back to Hartsfield...for a third time, and his sixth overall rehab visit.

Maximillian's relapses fit the classic profile of a person in recovery. The greatest vulnerability for relapse following treatment is the first 30 to 90 days after discharge. Most people who are completing addiction treatment walk a tightrope between sustained recovery and resumption of alcohol use. Over half will drink in the year following discharge from treatment. Between 25 and 35 percent of people who complete addiction treatment will be readmitted within a year, and 50 percent will be readmitted within four years.

Once he finished up his third course of detox and aftercare at Hartsfield, Maximillian made a pact with himself that he'd done his last stint in rehab. He was going to stand down his demons and crush them like ants.

Margaret, as she did during each rehab stint, went to his house and removed every ounce of alcohol before Maximillian could find it. She scoured the place. Not just the regular nooks and crannies, like the liquor cabinet, refrigerator, and closet, but places other people would never have looked. Under the bed. In his clothes hamper. In an old pair of boots. Next to a hat rack. And the most interesting place of all, inside a hollowed-out copy of the King James Bible.

Finding the Strength?

Back home in Chelsea, Maximillian found initial strength in his resolution not to drink. He vowed to replace time spent drinking with exercise. In one fell swoop, he had a delivery truck bring a Peloton bike and both rowing and elliptical machines. A man came to the house to measure his feet and put him on a bi-monthly subscription for new running shoes. And he bought a juicer, one that Margaret had researched on the Web as being "the easiest way to capture essential vitamins, minerals, and nutrients."

Maximillian wanted to get back to being the force that had taken him to the top of every place he'd ever worked. His securities firm wasn't floundering, but it wasn't seizing opportunities that many felt would secure its future. Maximillian's advisors told him that acquiring a business unit as a means to enter the U.S. market would make tremendous sense.

With his mind clear and body in better shape than it had been in years, Maximillian boarded a plane to New York. He was due to meet with executives from PlusTrade, a growing entity in the securities field known for being customer-focused and dedicated to solid research. Word was that the company was looking for a partner with whom it could pursue global business.

PlusTrade's executives treated Maximillian well. They took him to some of the city's best restaurants. They proved to be gracious hosts and mixed socializing with business. Maximillian interspersed looking at their financials with trips to Broadway and the Yankee Stadium. In all his journeys to the U.S., Maximillian had never been to a baseball game. He sat with the executives from PlusTrade in their box seats as the firm's CFO explained the intricacies of the game. Maximillian found the atmosphere stimulating, comparing fan reactions to the chants he heard at Chelsea games.

All the while, he somehow found the strength to stay away from liquor. People around him drank before dinner and with their meals, but he steadfastly refused.

After six days of observation, conversation, and examination, it looked like PlusTrade and SecureValue were on the verge of striking a deal. But with four hours left until Maximillian's plane was due to depart, he sensed a shift in tone. Only a few hours earlier, the PlusTrade execs had seemed eager to speak with him on just about anything. Now they seemed guarded and hesitant when speaking of the future. With a hearty handshake, the people at PlusTrade bid Maximillian adieu and sent him on his way to Kennedy Airport.

As he was waiting for his plane, which was running an hour late, he received a call from PlusTrade. The firm's CFO said any potential deal was off.

Maximillian felt like he'd been punched in the gut. He retreated to the business traveler's lounge, where he watched an American television channel devoted to business. The man at the anchor desk said the following:

"This just in. PlusTrade, the New York-based securities firm, has just inked a deal with Canadian banking giant Royal Trust. The deal calls for Royal Trust to acquire PlusTrade and all its assets for 2.3 billion dollars. PlusTrade executives say the deal is beneficial to their customers and will help Royal Trust make a substantial splash in the U.S. market."

"I've been duped!" thought Maximillian. "They played me for a stooge! A week in New York when all I did was act like a terrier in their dog-and-pony show...and what've I got to show for it? NOTHING!"

Maximillian then walked up to the bar.

"Whiskey, please. Rocks."

There it went - six months of sobriety down the tubes.

On the Plane

Maximillian boarded the Heathrow-bound jet. He had a window seat in first class. A man in a dark grey suit with his tie loosened sat across from him. The two nodded at each other in recognition and exchanged pleasantries.

"Good to be headed back," said the man in the dark grey suit.

"Right," responded Maximillian. "Long day. Long week, really."

The plane readied for takeoff, and all electronic devices had to be turned off. Then, the Captain applied maximum thrust to the four Rolls Royce engines, and with a mighty shove like a hurricane, they soared into the late afternoon sky. The two men, with nothing else seemingly to do, struck up a conversation.

"So what brings you to the States?" Maximillian asked.

"I'm a doctor," the man in the grey suit replied. "My name is John Horacio Harrow. Great to meet you. I was here on a conference about addiction medicine. I have a practice in Harley Street but go back and forth to the states about six times per year. Used to live here, and have licenses to practice in the U.K. and the U.S."

"You don't say?" responded Maximillian, somewhat marveled. "That's funny. I have a license to drink in both the U.K. and the U.S."

The two men, who clearly enjoyed the art of conversation and found it a welcome diversion to the transatlantic flight, seemed able to talk about anything. The subject of the Chelsea football club must have taken up to an hour itself. Maximillian had three whiskeys during that portion of things.

The subject of restaurants popped up, too. Both men, despite their comfortable livings, were fascinated not so much with highly-rated, high-priced establishments, but places where you could get "the best" of something for what they would consider virtually "shillings".

"Best place to get breakfast?" Maximillian asked John.

"Easy," John replied. "The Bumpkin in South Kensington.

The fried breakfast really is cracking. And if you need an early lunch, try Abruzzi's on King Street the roast beef and steaks are the dog's bollocks. How about this...best dim sum?"

"That's a breeze," Maximillian shot back. "Yauatcha's in Soho. The sauce makes the filling just stand on its head. Then, you move over to one of their patisseries. They're brilliant."

Their conversation about food lasted for about another hour. It also gave Maximillian a chance to order three more whiskeys.

Next, they moved on to talk about furnishings.

"I furnished my whole flat with things I found at the Portobello Market," Maximillian said. "Great antiques there. My assistant, Margaret, helped me out. She also turned me on to one of the fruit stands there. She made me declare every first Monday of the month 'Healthy Monday' at the office, so I usually stop there on the way in to get stuff for everyone."

"Oh, I love the place," John said. "I sometimes spend whatever lunch hour I take wandering around and eating. Sometimes my nurses take up a collection and bring back full meals for everyone to pick at during the day."

After Maximillian had another two whiskeys, talk turned back to their lines of work.

"So, I never asked what you were doing in New York?" queried John.

"Kind of an odd story, really," replied Maximillian. "I own a securities firm, and we were looking to go global with the right kind of situation. So I went and took a hard look at an American firm. Spent seven days with them. Nice chaps, really. They treated me like I was their own 'Uncle Nije'; taking me places, filling my belly with good stuff, showing me their books.

"But...I don't know...something happened," Maximillian groused. "I mean, one minute they're happy as Larry and the next it's like they all got a memo to put a sock in it. Looked like we were about to shake on things, and then it was like they had to see a man about a dog. If that wasn't bad enough, just after I get a call at the airport that the deal was off, I turn on the telly and see they've signed on with Royal Trust in Canada. Bloody 'ell! I never felt like such a tube!"

John couldn't help but notice that Maximillian's mood took a real swing during that conversation. One moment he had been chatty and happy; the next, it was like he'd gotten the hump.

"Miss," Maximillian called out to the flight attendant as he pointed to his empty glass. "I need another one of these! I've gotta go siphon the python, so that should give you enough time to bring me another. And make it a double! I've just lost the deal of a lifetime!"

By the time he returned to his seat, the flight attendant was waiting for him.

"Sir," she said. "I've been told by the captain that this is your last one. I can't have you going off your trolley before we get to Heathrow. So please, do me a favor and don't get in a paddy before we land."

"OK, love," Maximillian responded. "Will do."

As an aside to John, Maximillian remarked, "She's got some nice baps, she does."

Most people would be taken aback by such behavior; many would cower away with a look on their face saying, "I'm not with that guy." John, on the other hand, could spot the behavior for what it was - addiction.

After about 10 minutes of silence, he decided it was a good idea to present Maximillian with his card.

"Listen, mate," John said. "Let me give you this. It's my card. It's got my cell number on the back. I'm a guy who treats many blokes who drink a bit. A lot of them have come to me in a bad way - about to lose their jobs, homes, wives, and kids; the full monty. And I've been able to help get them back on the right path. It's a bit off the beaten path for you as I am in Miami, but just give me a couple of weeks to set things right. The clinic is called Privée Clinics."

"I have wanted to cut back for some time," Maximillian said. "Been to AA. Been to rehab. Once tried hypnosis and then acupuncture. Nothing seems to work. Something happens, and no matter how much I try, after a few months... bloody 'ell! I'm back in the big house!"

"So has anybody ever offered you medicines to help control your cravings for drinks?" asked John.

"No," said Maximillian. "Never. Each rehab place I've been to tells me that using drugs to stay off drink doesn't solve anything. They said it's like substituting one drug for another. When I went to AA, they said anybody who got off drinking by using medicine was nothing more than a dry drunk."

"Things have changed, mate," John said. "That's 1950s thinking is what that is. Old wives' tales and that sort of thing. You've got to get your brain right again. It's that simple. Please, give me a call. I can help get you started."

Signature Scene: The Card

Outside the terminal, the air had that thin, metallic smell of aviation fuel and rain. Maximillian walked a few steps ahead of John as if distance could keep him safe. In his pocket, the card felt heavier than paper should.

He waited until John disappeared into the flow of passengers before pulling it out. A name. A number written in neat, practical ink. An offer that wasn't a lecture or a threat - just a door left unlocked.

Maximillian had spent his adult life translating risk into profit. He could read markets the way some people read faces. But the problem in his chest and the problem in his drinking did not behave like markets. They did not correct themselves. They did not respond to confidence. They only responded to truth, and truth was the one thing he had been avoiding with professional skill.

He imagined dialing the number and saying, *I need help.* The words tasted like weakness. He could already hear the old voice in his head - sharp, amused, cruel - telling him to handle it the way he handled everything else: privately, efficiently, without witnesses.

By the time he reached his car, he'd built a compromise. He would let Margaret call. He would become "a friend." The lie felt absurd as soon as he formed it, but it also felt familiar. It was the same bargain he made with alcohol: just enough honesty to ease the pressure, not enough to change the story.

Still Not Quite Fessing Up

"He seemed like a nice chap, Margaret," Maximillian explained to his faithful, long-time assistant. "But I don't know. I don't want to come across as too forward or that I'm a complete rat-arsed loony. Can't you call him?"

"What'll I say?" Margaret asked.

"Tell him you have 'this friend' who's been drinking a lot lately," Maximillian instructed. "Tell him he's basically a nice fellow, but he's having some trouble keeping sober. Ask him what kind of drugs he puts people on and what happens to them when they go on that stuff."

As Margaret spoke with Dr. Harrow, Maximillian loomed behind her.

"No," John said. "It's not like that at all. It's not an addicting drug. People take it. It does what it has to do. I want to take a sample of their blood, and if the genetics match, we can consider an ultra-low-dose ondansetron approach that has been explored in precision-minded clinical research. It remains investigational in many settings, and the science is still evolving—but for the right person, under the right supervision, it may reduce craving and help the brain regain traction. If the person qualifies and is willing to try, I can help guide them—carefully, ethically, and with the data in mind."

Margaret then signed up her "friend" for an appointment with John. Knowing Maximillian's schedule by heart, she signed him up for the following Tuesday afternoon at his clinic in Miami.

The Science of Ultra-low-dose Ondansetron

Ondansetron is a 5-HT3 receptor antagonist. 5-HT3

receptors in the brain are co-localized with dopamine pathways. Dopamine pathways in the orbitofrontal cortex and mesolimbic areas (in lay terms, if you stick your fingers up your nose and run it by the side of your head to about a few inches before you reach the beginning of your neck) are considered to be the neurobiological substrate through which addiction is expressed. That pathway is associated with other brain regions that are associated with learned fear, memories, and the expression of behaviors. At its simplest conception, what you perceive (alcohol or the abused drug) is routed into what you think, which is modified by how you feel and your memories, and results in how you actually behave. In normal behaviors, this reinforcing or rewarding pathway helps to consolidate behaviors, especially natural reinforcers such as food and sex, and give them a pleasurable or habit-forming effect. When an individual becomes addicted, these pathways are “hijacked” such that the reward salience (i.e., what is paramount to be reinforced by the brain) is the use of more alcohol or drugs.

Preclinical and pharmacobehavioral studies suggest that blockade of serotonin-3 receptors will influence the dopamine reward system activated by alcohol, thereby decreasing dopamine release and attenuating craving for alcohol (Johnson, BA et al., 2002; Lovinger, DM, 1999).

Early clinical studies found that the efficacy of ultra-low-dose ondansetron is limited to certain subgroups of the alcohol-dependent population and suggested the differential effect could be predicted based on the age of onset of alcoholism, an indistinct concept likely confounded by genetic, regional and ethnic differences (Johnson, BA et al., 2000;

Kranzler, HR et al., 2003). Recent research suggests the variable effect may be predictable based on molecular mechanism of ultra-low-dose ondansetron action and individual subject genotype of key genes in the serotonin system (Enoch, MA et al., 2010; Johnson, BA et al., 2011).

Success in Phase II studies, and progression to Phase III

In a pivotal Phase 2b clinical trial, Prof. Dr. Bankole Johnson and his team discovered that ultra-low-dose ondansetron, the active pharmaceutical agent in AD04, showed a statistically significant difference between ondansetron and placebo for both the primary endpoint and secondary endpoint. The differences were: a reduction in the severity of drinking measured in drinks per drinking day (1.71 drinks/drinking day; p=0.0042), and a reduction in the frequency of drinking measured in days of abstinence/no drinking (11.56%; p=0.0352), respectively. Additionally, and importantly, the Phase 2b results showed a significant decrease in the percentage of heavy drinking days (11.08%; p=0.0445) with a "heavy drinking day" defined as a day with four (4) or more alcoholic drinks for women or five (5) or more alcoholic drinks for men consumed in the same day. The target genotypes were polymorphic variants at the serotonin transporter (*SLC6A4*-LL/TT) and the serotonin receptor (*HTR3A*-rs1150226-AG, *HTR3A*-rs1176713-GG, and *HTR3B*-rs17614942-AC) in a 4-marker but 5 genotype panel.

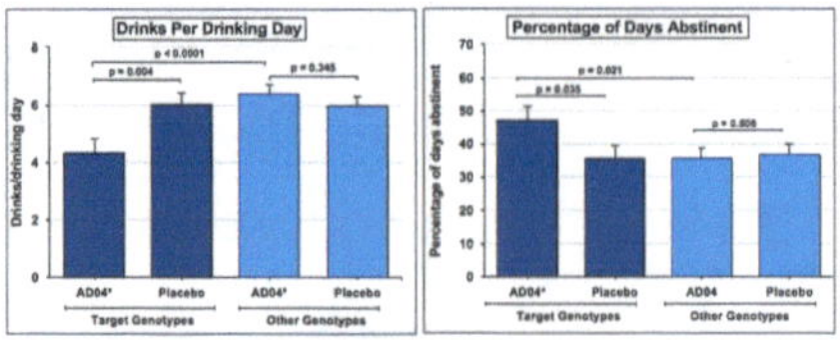

Figure: Ultra-low-dose ondansetron - a precision-medicine approach.

Ultra-low-dose ondansetron has been explored as a precision-minded approach to alcohol use disorder. One development program built around genetic target profiles (Adial Pharmaceuticals' AD04) has been investigated in Phase 3 clinical testing. As with all therapeutics discussed in this book, nothing here is a prescription, endorsement, or regulatory claim; approvals and indications evolve, and clinicians should consult current prescribing information and regulatory guidance.

A short video of how ultra-low-dose ondansetron may work to treat alcohol use disorder can be viewed.

Getting Maximillian Back on Track

When Maximillian met with Dr. John Horacio Harrow, he had been drinking for the better part of three weeks since the deal with PlusTrade fell through. The first thing Dr. Harrow did was take blood and urine samples from Maximillian. Dr. Harrow was astonished to learn that Maximillian had the genetics to qualify for a trial of ultra-low-dose ondansetron. How lucky was that? Only 34.6% of people qualify, but there were signs that he might; such as drinking from a very early age under pressure (a feature called early-onset alcohol use disorder), a family history of excessive drinking, and a notable level of anxiety, which was easy to miss because of his bravado.

Next, Dr. Harrow negotiated with the Company that marketed ultra-low-dose ondansetron for some of the medicine for "compassionate use", and they obliged. Dr. Harrow began his treatment of Maximillian, not telling him to stop drinking immediately, but to set a target goal of weekly reductions. Dr. Harrow would monitor his progress through speaking with him, and also taking serial samples of his blood to measure the biological component of the genetic marker called mRNA. That was it! No detox, no night sweats, and no forced sobriety.

Maximillian tolerated the ultra-low dose ondansetron well, with only an occasional mild headache. Indeed, he felt, at times, like he was taking nothing at all.

Maximillian coupled his ultra-low-dose ondansetron intake with targeted sessions of Brief Behavioral Compliance Enhancement Treatment (BBCET), and after two weeks of staying in a hotel in Miami, and seeing Dr. Harrow every other day, flew back to NYC.

Dr. Harrow assured Maximilian that in-between his visits to Miami, he would work with his local doctor in NYC to keep him on track, and also, meet with him regularly by video conference on Zoom™

Finally, Maximillian started to get a handle on his drinking, and his impulsive personality that seemed to trigger the drinking seemed to get better, too, almost all by itself. As he started to recover, Dr. Harrow added both lifestyle discussions with him and targeted Cognitive Behavioral Treatment (CBT) with a psychologist to his treatment to give him the skills to prevent further relapses. Maximilian gained an understanding of why he never married. He had regular appointments with Dr. Harrow - every two weeks at first, monthly after that. His blood work was analyzed regularly, and by the time he hit the five-month time point, his metabolic profile was back to near normal, indicating that the damage he had been doing to his liver and kidneys were coming under control. Maximillian did not mind the constant traveling to see Dr. Harrow in Miami. After all, what was a 2-hour ride on NetJets compared to long transatlantic flights? Those office visits were "precious" to Maximillian as it allowed him to "reset" his life and become more educated about the dangers of alcohol use disorder.

Ultra-low-dose ondansetron helped Maximillian get past that magic six-month plateau of sobriety. It gave his brain a chance to essentially rewire itself and recover.

After one year of sobriety, Maximillian met John Horacio Harrow for breakfast at The Bumpkin in London. The two continued the easy conversations they'd had in Dr. Harrow's office. Soccer, cars, and social issues were among the topics. But Maximillian introduced a totally unexpected subject.

"I got engaged," Maximillian said. "To Margaret! Save a Sunday next April for the wedding."

"Crickey!" John shot back. "Congratulations, old duck!"

"She was always there right under my nose," Maximillian said. "Through all the time I've been trying to stop drinking, the rehabs, the daft episodes; she's always looked out for me. I mean, how many people really get to be married to their best mate?"

Review

Maximillian's pattern of drinking and rehab

Maximillian had been a heavy drinker for several years, especially since he was an adolescent.

He attended rehab six times.

He had trouble staying sober past the four-month point following rehab stints.

He had a family history of alcohol use disorder.

He had notable social anxiety.

How did Maximillian learn about ultra-low-dose ondansetron?

On his flight back to London, Maximillian ended up sitting next to a doctor who specialized in addiction medicine.

The doctor witnessed Maximillian's addictive behavior firsthand.

His doctor took blood tests.

-Results revealed that Maximillian had the right genetic profile, found in 34.6% of those with European or Hispanic descent.

-He found that taking ultra-low-dose ondsnetron made sense in an individual with potentially other significant health problems due to his length of drinking.

His doctor negotiated with Maximillian on a program to reduce his drinking and eventually stop.

Once that goal had been reached, Maximillian could enter into a more lifestyle-based and cognitive treatment to improve his skills to prevent relapse.

Why was Maximillian a good candidate for ultra-low-dose ondansetron?

He had the right genetic profile to gain the maximum benefit from the treatment.

He was not interested in more rehabs or "go it alone" treatments.

He had social anxiety, and as ultra-low dose ondansetron is an anxiolytic, decreasing his anxiety would increase his ability to recover and prevent relapse.

He was impulsive, suffered mood swings, all of which gave Dr. Harrow a clue that he had abnormality within the serotonin system, which is involved with mood regulation in the brain.

How does ultra-low-dose ondansetron work?

Ultra-low dose ondansetron is a specific blocker of the serotonin-3 (5-HT3) receptor.

Ondansetron is currently used for the treatment of emesis, but the lowest dose presently available commercially is 12 times bigger than the dose required to treat Maximillian.

Giving Maximillian the currently available dose would have worsened his symptoms or had no effect. This was not discussed in the story but has been demonstrated by research. Thus, the only dose that would work could only have been obtained from the Company licensed to manufacture and market that dose - Adial Pharmaceuticals.

Ultra-low-dose ondansetron has few side effects. These side-effects are principally headache, constipation, and fatigue. Indeed, so few are the side effects of ultra-low-dose ondansetron, that in comparative studies with placebo, some side effects were more common in the placebo group.

Psychosocial support with ultra-low dose ondansetron focused on BBCET - also developed by Prof Dr. Bankole

Johnson, and for longer-term relapse prevention, CBT was administered to teach relapse prevention skills.

Maximillian's Treatment and follow-up

He had regular appointments at the Miami clinic for the first two weeks as an outpatient, and then this progressed to a mixture of videoconferencing and return-visits to the facility.

Life-style management discussions also were introduced to Maximillian by his doctor in Miami.

His blood work was analyzed regularly.

By the time he was five months sober, his metabolic profile was under control, and he had reversed much of the physical damage of his years of excessive alcohol consumption.

Ultra-low dose ondansetron helped him to achieve and maintain sobriety longer than he ever had and gave his brain a chance to essentially "rewire" itself and recover.

* * *

Signature Reflection: The Frequent Flyer

Maximillian lives in motion because stillness is where the questions wait. The story reframes "high-functioning" as a delay, not a defense. Precision care - right treatment, right patient - becomes a new kind of humility: admitting that biology matters, and that it can be guided.

If you remember one thing: precision replaces shame with strategy.

- The dragon's disguise: ambition that makes self-destruction look like drive.

- The turning point: individualized treatment that matches the person's biology and pattern of use.
- A practice to try: track your triggers for one week - time of day, emotion, setting - then change one variable on purpose.

Clinical lens: ondansetron's role in alcohol use disorder is linked to serotonin signaling and is most relevant to specific patient profiles. The broader principle is the Signature Series core: personalize care.

The Star Teacher

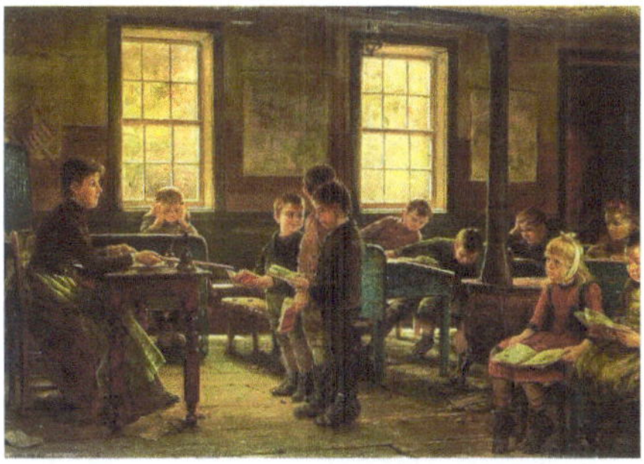

The image above is: Country-school painting - Edward Lamson Henry.

Edward Lamson Henry's country-school painting holds a gentle nostalgia: warm wood, attentive faces, learning as a shared ritual. Henry was known for American genre scenes and for depicting rural life in the long shadow of the Civil War. The image suggests stability - the kind Abby Jensen works tirelessly to provide, even as her private life begins to fray.

Acamprosate, the medication featured in this story, is one way to make early sobriety physiologically tolerable by helping rebalance glutamatergic signaling after abstinence. But the first medicine is often permission: to ask for help without losing dignity. When Dragons Kill, they sometimes do it in silence.

Once each marking period, she had students dress in period clothing to bring specific events to life: colonial attire for Thomas Jefferson, Civil War regalia for Gettysburg, industrial-revolution roles from factory workers to bankers, and spectators at the March on Washington waiting to hear Dr. Martin Luther King speak.

Abby had a sharp sense of humor and could meet twelve-year-olds where they lived. She also took the craft of teaching seriously enough to know that love wasn't enough; good teachers wear many hats.

Harrow's Field Note: The Quietest Addictions

History teacher Abby Jensen was the kind of adult many sixth-graders said they wanted to become. She didn't just teach history - she inhabited it. Even her colleagues called her their "very own Doris Kearns Goodwin," in homage to the noted historian.

Once per marking period, she had her students dress up in period clothing to bring specific events to life. On one occasion, they came in colonial attire to cap off their studies of Thomas Jefferson. Another time it was in Civil War regalia, to commemorate the Battle of Gettysburg. Once, her students donned garb representing the spectrum of people involved in the industrial revolution - from foremen and factory workers to bankers and inventors. Still another time, they dressed as spectators at the March on Washington, waiting to hear Dr. Martin Luther King speak.

Abby had a sharp sense of humor and could relate to 12-year-old kids in ways that other teachers simply couldn't. That may have been because she took the art of teaching very seriously. She knew that getting through to them took more than just loving kids; it meant embracing the idea that good teachers often need to wear several hats.

Those hats include being a communicator, disciplinarian, evaluator, classroom manager, counselor, decision-maker, role model, and surrogate parent. Many of those roles were not taught in her undergraduate or master's classes; she had picked them up from experience, other teachers, mentors, and her mom and dad, who had both been teachers.

Her dad had always been an inspiration. He was the kind of man who, alongside his job as a high school science teacher, was active in the community. When it came to winding down from all that, she remembered him almost decompressing at the end of the day over a glass of scotch. As she grew older, Abby began to realize that the one glass of scotch actually grew to like two or three on most nights.

Lifelong Learning

Abby's first year of teaching barely resembled her subsequent years at Central Middle School. Her lesson plans were meticulous, and her conversations with students were amiable, but something felt dry and stiff about the way history was being presented through textbooks.

Relying on academic narratives, Abby found, was not

bringing her passion for history alive. She wanted to light a fire for history in her students and longed to tap into the experiences she had gained while her parents indulged her interest in history. They had taken Abby and her brother to historical sites every summer. Her favorite trip had been their tour of Civil War battlegrounds, including Gettysburg, Antietam, Harper's Ferry, and sites in Virginia's Shenandoah Valley.

Following a conversation with Jane Matthews, a science teacher two years her senior at Central, Abby decided it would be a good idea to join a teacher's networking and peer group.

"You think I came up with the idea of separating kids into protons and electrons by myself?" Jane, a group member, asked. "I got it from a guy in my middle school teacher's group. This guy who's been teaching for 23 years up in Brighton told me about it. He said it was just a little thing he figured out to keep his kids engaged. He'd been doing it for 21 years before I met him, and he thought it was part of the reason he'd been named 'favorite teacher' by kids in his school 14 times."

The conversation with Jane led Abby to join a group of history teachers at the Western Counties Middle School Teachers Group. She formed a close relationship with four other teachers. There was Suzy, who'd been teaching for six years at a middle school a few towns over; Phil, who'd left a Wall Street life 10 years prior to get his teaching degree, and now had seven years under his belt; Sharon, out of college for two years and teaching at a school in a blue-collar area; and Jack, a guy who'd been enjoying life as a teacher for 25 years.

Over time, Suzy, Sharon, and Abby became close. They would go to dinner sometimes or meet for a drink at a tavern located where none of the parents from their schools would find them. Abby enjoyed her time conversing with Phil as well, finding that his disdain of the "profits-over-people" philosophy he'd seen on Wall Street still drove his desire to teach kids about mistakes of the past. But it was Jack that Abby looked up to the most.

Jack had the look of a favorite professor; he sported cardigan sweaters and loafers. His hair (what was left of it) covered his head in a partial comb-over. He favored argyle socks and pleated pants because, he said, his wife loved them.

"Can you tell whether you have a particularly disinterested group of kids just by looking at them on the first day of school?" Abby asked Jack.

"Sometimes," he answered. "It might take a day or so till you gather their reputations from the teachers they had last year, but I've had that sense early on. When you get that inkling, you have to start thinking about what you're going to do differently that year. You need to find ways to augment and even deviate from your lesson plans."

A year or so later, Abby asked Jack whether he thought kids were just bored with learning.

"Kids are changing," Jack said. "They can sit in front of the TV and watch 100 channels of drivel, play video games, or stare at a computer screen. Some of them think history is last year's pop sensation. Sometimes you gotta be a little foolish to get their attention, but they'll get your drift after a while.

Most of 'em can tell you're trying and 'keeping it real.' They'll respond."

By her third year at Central, Abby was coming in dressed as George Washington on every first day of school, complete with a set of yellowed dentures. She'd always ask students their names with an accent she'd picked up from watching the movie *1776* one too many times. After a few years, the buzz on how she was expected to dress for the first day of school was palpable. As kids lined up in the gymnasium waiting to be dispatched to their classes, she'd make her way through the crowd asking whether anyone had "seen a cherry tree" or anyone was "telling a lie."

Building a Home Life

Abby met Steve Marshall at a wedding not long after she got the job at Central. Steve was three years her elder and had joined an accounting firm after getting his master's degree. When he sat next to Abby, he casually mentioned that he could help her out with her taxes. She responded by saying that she had decided not to pay her taxes and would be dumping the King's tea into Boston Harbor in protest. Steve got the reference, and their romance blossomed from there.

Abby and Steve were married about two years after they met, during her second summer break as a teacher. It gave them time to take a two-week honeymoon cruise to Western Europe. She suggested that they spend most of their time on land visiting castles and ancient forts, and he was all-too-happy to oblige.

Upon returning from their honeymoon, they took up residence in a newly constructed two-bedroom townhouse. Steve had purchased the place with the idea that it would appreciate in value over the next few years. And Abby didn't mind the spacious master bedroom, kitchen with new appliances, and neutral carpet. She surprised Steve one late July day by accenting one wall of their bedroom a sedate shade of burgundy. Despite never having seen such a vibrant color indoors, he had no objection to her painting the rest of the townhouse.

Since Steve's tax seasons were usually busy, Abby scheduled two classes during spring semesters en route to obtaining her master's degree in teaching. The school district was picking up the tab for her education, under the agreement that she'd complete the program within five years. Knowing that Steve would be working late most nights between mid-January and April 15, Abby thought she could put her "alone" time to good use.

Support from Peers and Family

The effect of the four history teachers whom Abby leaned on from the Western Counties Teachers Group was palpable. She used their support to continually adapt her approach to teaching and passed along her ideas to other teachers at Central. The support of her peer group helped her combat the emotional drain she felt on certain days in the classroom.

While the support of peers is important, some experts feel that relationships outside of school are just as important for helping teachers fulfill their professional duties. Teachers who spend time with family and friends are more likely to return to the classroom mentally and emotionally refreshed. And that balance of personal and professional lives helps them grow in all areas of life.

Of the teachers in her peer group, Suzy, Sharon, and Phil

spoke of the strong relationships they still had with their parents. And Jack, even though his parents had died five years earlier, spoke of the way he had fished with his father until the man's 85th birthday and how he and his wife had played board games with his mother, who remained sharp and active until her death at age 86.

Jack, Sharon, and Phil talked about how their kids helped them become better teachers and people. Jack told Abby that when his kids were growing up, he and his wife made sure they'd sit together for meals and have in-depth conversations. Even if he sat there and just listened, Jack always felt they were at least providing him with some kind of insight on how kids think.

Both Suzy and Phil, though their kids were younger, stated that being a parent helped them deal with kids better. The experience of raising kids had made them much more tolerant, patient, and understanding.

And even Sharon, who felt that she was "too young for kids," spoke about the support she'd gained from a strong marriage.

"My marriage makes me a better teacher," Sharon said. "It makes me feel like I don't have any serious personal issues that would make me really unhappy."

Abby and Steve had discussed having children, especially after Abby had completed her master's program. By age 28, she was ready. By age 29, she was chomping at the bit.

But Steve always seemed to have other things going on that provided reasons not to have kids. He was "getting close to partner" at his accounting firm. Going to see clients involved "too much traveling" to have kids. He was "so involved in other things" that he wasn't sure when he could sit down and figure things out.

Something had changed in their marriage. And by the time she was 31, Abby found herself alone many nights with a big glass of wine, reading such books as *Mornings on Horseback*, a story about Teddy Roosevelt.

A Great Wine, a Great Time

Abby had developed a taste for wine after a trip she and Steve had taken to California's Napa and Sonoma regions. Having been more of a beer drinker beforehand, the winery tours provided her with an appreciation for everything that went into winemaking, and for detecting the complexities in each bottle. Learning the challenges faced by wine producers, and the chronicles of each winery fit in well with her passion for history.

She enjoyed detecting the subtle mint and eucalyptus flavors that characterized a cabernet sauvignon. She could also tell when a "cab" had grapes that were picked too early because there was always too much green bell pepper flavor.

She learned to appreciate a light-bodied pinot grigio. Their bouquets with hints of pear, apple, or melon provided a great balance to the crisp, refreshing taste with flavors of pepper and arugula pushing through.

But it was the more common pinot noir that remained her favorite. She sought out pinots of medium body with aromas of black cherry, raspberry, or currant. She'd embraced the character of pinot, "a wine so romantic, with a perfume so voluptuous, an edge so sweet, and a punch so powerful that it resembled the essence of falling in love," according to one critic. She also enjoyed other characterizations of pinot noir as “sex in a glass” or “a seductive yet fickle mistress.”

Abby prided herself in being able to pick great wines that tasted like they were much more expensive. Friends knew they could leave the task of choosing the wine to her, whether it was out on the town or at home for a small gathering. She kept her eyes open for wine sales at some of the larger liquor outlets in her area, making sure to buy cases when opportunities arose.

Taking Stock and Coming Up Empty

By the time Abby reached her 33rd birthday, it was clear that her marriage was on the wane. Steve had grown distant and seemed even more married to his work. She remembered the fun guy she had fallen in love with back at that wedding but didn’t seem to recognize him anymore.

While she continued to pour her heart and soul into teaching, her nights alone were becoming increasingly blurry. A big glass of wine turned into two big glasses of wine.

When Steve announced that he thought it was time for him and Abby to separate, two big glasses turned into three or four.

She had had conversations with her mother about the challenges of marriage. Those talks made her confident that she could navigate any rough waters. Being persistent with Steve, she thought, would help fulfill her destiny as that old married couple that people see sitting on a porch swing, discussing how their grandchildren were growing.

But now, her crumbled marriage made her feel like a failure. On top of that, it felt like the support system around her was falling apart.

Abby's dad had taken ill and, within two months, passed away. He had developed pancreatic cancer, which was first diagnosed when it was already in an advanced stage. The man who had inspired her so much was gone. She took two weeks off from school, during which time she helped plan a funeral, accepted friends and family at a two-day wake, buried her father, and retreated to the privacy of her husband-less townhouse. Jack, Suzy, Sharon, and Phil came to the funeral. But she found that not as many teachers from Central had made it. A few stopped by during the wake, as did the Central principal, but some of the younger teachers she had mentored did not. Their absence weighed on her mind.

Those two weeks gave her a bit too much time alone; it seemed. And four big glasses of wine per night turned into one more in the morning, two more at lunch, and one in the afternoon. There became no distinction between dinnertime and her nightly ritual. Wine with dinner turned into wine with dessert and prime-time TV.

Realizing that she was due to return to school in two days, she decided to sober up a bit and cut down on her wine consumption. By Sunday, she was down to just three big glasses.

Upon her return to school, everyone offered sympathy, from her students to the janitors. She felt some comfort in their words, but the emptiness caused by the loss of her father seemed like an unwelcome guest who didn't want to leave.

During her first week back, Abby began screening for her students the Ken Burns Civil War documentary. The epic piece consisted of nine episodes lasting 10 hours total. It was one of her favorite pieces of storytelling, and she built up class anticipation for the film over the course of the school year.

On Friday of that first week back, during the third episode that featured narratives on Stonewall Jackson and the Seven Days Battles, Abby asked her student-teacher to keep an eye on her class while she took care of some things. She used the opportunity to sneak out to her car...and pull out a bottle of pinot noir from under her seat.

Signature Scene: Parking Lot Confessional

Abby's keys bit into her palm as she crossed the parking lot. The hallway noise - lockers, laughter, a teacher calling a name - faded behind her as she slid into her car and shut the door. For a few seconds, she just sat there with both hands on the steering wheel, breathing like she'd run a mile.

On the screen in her mind, Ken Burns' documentary kept rolling: Stonewall Jackson, the Seven Days Battles, men marching toward consequences they could not fully imagine. Abby stared at her own reflection in the rearview mirror and thought, not for the first time, that grief was a kind of war - one that kept drafting you even when you wanted to surrender.

The bottle was where she'd left it, wrapped in a sweater like contraband. She hated that she'd planned it. She hated that she'd needed to. The first twist of the cap sounded too loud in the sealed car.

She lifted the bottle and paused, eyes closed. Somewhere inside the building, her students were waiting. They trusted her. They believed she had control. Abby took a swallow anyway, chasing a moment of numbness the way she used to chase a spark of inspiration.

The wine hit her stomach and did what it always did: it quieted the panic for a heartbeat. Then the panic returned, sharper, because now it had company - shame. Abby wiped her mouth with the back of her hand, stared at the school doors, and told herself she would be better tomorrow. She said it like a prayer, and it frightened her how automatic the prayer had become.

She took a few swigs and then was scared when she imagined what it would look like if she were ever caught:

'Cops Find Teacher Drunk at School,' the headline would scream. Or *'33-Year-Old Middle School Teacher Busted with Bottle of Pinot to Her Lips.'*

(AP) _ A Central Middle School teacher has been arrested for allegedly teaching while drunk. History teacher, Abby Jensen, was taken to the county jail on Friday afternoon and booked for investigation of felony child endangerment.

Administrators at Central Middle School told the county sheriff that the teacher was apparently intoxicated on campus. Another teacher at the school, on condition of anonymity, said that would probably explain Jensen's propensity for dressing up like Abraham Lincoln in recent weeks.

School district Superintendent, Ted McNeil, said there was never a threat to Jensen's sixth-grade students. Jensen has been placed on leave.

The Cumulative Effect

Abby figured she needed to be more discreet with her drinking methods. But as time went on, she became less discriminating about her wine.

Having been a connoisseur of wines in the $10-to-$15 range, she had given up those up for the easy fix of something referred to as "Two-Dollar Dan." Two-Dollar Dan was actually 64 ounces of a red wine blend that came in a paper bottle and sold for $2 at a big box retailer. Some wine critics even called it an "excellent value" buy.

The effect of the abundant cheap wine on Abby was becoming more evident. Where she used to be among the first teachers at school in the morning, she was now among the last. Where she used to be bright and attentive, even when watching a documentary with her class, she was now lightly snoozing. Where she had been active with the debate club, she now asked that the team's co-coach take on more responsibility.

Finally, Central Middle School's principal, Art Riegel, called her into his office.

"Abby," Art said, "I don't want to come down too hard on you. I know you've been through a lot lately, but you know I have a responsibility to the kids and the parents of Central. It's pretty obvious to your colleagues and to me that something is up with you that needs straightening out."

Abby burst into tears. She had feared this was coming. She could only blurt out, "I'm sorry" about 10 times.

"This stuff does happen," said Art. "We all work in a tough profession. It's not all fun and games. Kids are becoming more challenging every day. They all seem to know 'too much.' But I know you're a great teacher. The kids love you. You've proven that time and time again. So I want you to get better.

"This is what I'm going to suggest," Art continued. "Go on over to the district office and talk with Perry in HR. We've got decent benefits through the state that can help you take care of things. Whatever time off you need I'm sure we can arrange for it. We're close enough to summer, so maybe we can get around things through the end of the school year and get you back by the start of next year."

Sobering Up

Abby's benefits covered 10 days of medical rehab and a 28-day stay for in-patient counseling. She decided to attend Majestic Shores Rehabilitation Hospital, named for its location near the convergence of two giant reservoirs.

In her first days after entering rehab, Abby experienced headaches like never before. The center was providing the drug, Klonopin, to ease withdrawal symptoms, but who knows how bad it would have been without that help. The staff was keeping an eye on her for any signs of delirium tremens, sometimes called "the DTs." The DTs involve sudden and severe mental or neurological changes characterized by excitement, fear, hallucinations, rapid mood changes, and seizures.

In Abby's second week of in-patient rehab, the members of her teaching group came to visit. She'd never been so happy to see their faces.

"Well, you look better," Sharon said. "We were pretty worried about you there for a while."

"I do feel better," Abby said. "I guess you really never

realize how so much wine can make you feel weighed down when you're just trying to carry yourself around on a daily basis."

"This kind of stuff happens to the best of us," Phil said. "I used to work with someone on Wall Street who was a great guy, but had problems dealing with pressure. He used to drink bourbon a lot, until one day they found him slumped over his desk with a glass sitting inches from his nose. Last I heard he got some help and got back to work."

"I don't know how many of us would have held up in your situation," Jack said. "Steve just up and leaves town without saying much, and then your dad dies. I can't say that wouldn't have driven me to lose control.

"And Phil's right," he continued. "It can happen to the best of us. I know a few people who are recovering alcoholics - teachers, actually. Things got to them - budget cuts, tough school districts, bad class assignments. But they bounced back. They all took the time to straighten up and regain their resolve about reaching kids the way they used to."

"Aw jeez," Abby responded. "Jack, you always know the right thing to say."

"To be honest," Suzy said, "I have some idea of what you're going through. By my second year out of college, I was acting like I was still in college. I was hitting the bottle pretty hard.

"But my dad sat me down and had a really serious talk with me," Suzy continued. "He kept a really close eye on me for a while and made me go talk to our family doctor. The doc told me about signs of alcohol abuse and that I was on the borderline of being an alcoholic. I don't know what happened, but by the time I was 25, I guess I'd had enough. I mean, you know, we've been together, and you've seen me drink, but I just don't have the desire to go beyond two glasses of wine."

At the end of their visit, Abby's peer group pledged to help her out in any way they could.

By the time she finished her rehab stint, she was ready to embrace summer vacation. She had planned to use her time off to go on short trips with her mom and maybe visit some friends from college. Abby decided to attend Alcoholics Anonymous meetings early in the morning, just before most attendees would need to leave for work. She figured it would give her a chance to start her day right and tackle her problem before other things got in the way.

Falling Down

About two weeks after joining AA, Abby had a conversation with Suzy that made her heart sink. Suzy's husband had accepted a new job in Florida, and her family would be moving there in July. Abby wished Suzy the best, but she felt sadness in knowing that a key member of her support team wouldn't be around much anymore.

As low as she felt when Suzy announced she was moving, nothing would prepare her for the depths she was about to experience. As she was preparing to travel with her mom, she received a phone call from Jack's wife, Ellen.

"Abby," she sobbed into the phone, "I hate to tell you this. But Jack died yesterday. He had a heart attack - a massive coronary. There was nothing that could save him. He may have been gone even before the paramedics came to the house."

"Oh, God!" Abby screamed. "Oh, that's terrible! Oh, I feel

horrible! I hope you guys are okay. When...when's the funeral?"

"On Saturday at St. Nick's on Valley Road," Ellen said. "Given everything that's happened, we're managing. It will take a while to sink in."

"Listen," Ellen said, "I know you've had some problems lately, but I'm sure Jack would want you to be safe and get as much help as you can. He used to tell me how much he enjoyed passing things on to you and just loved watching you develop as a teacher. So, we'd love to see you on Saturday, and please be strong."

"Thank you," Abby said. "I'll be there. And you be strong too."

"There it goes," Abby thought. "First, Steve, then my dad, then Suzy. Now...my biggest pillar of support is gone. What am I gonna do?"

Abby tried to hold it together for a few days. She promised she wouldn't give in to the temptation to drink, but it was too hard. She visited the local liquor store and bought two bottles of pinot noir. She paid $10 for one bottle that had a barnyard scene on the label and $7.99 for the second bottle, this one with a nice abstract painting pasted on. The two bottles lasted her two days.

She made it to Jack's funeral and kept herself together while sitting with Sharon, Phil, and Suzy, whose house had already been packed up for the big move. The four went to the cemetery and then back to Jack and Ellen's house to pay their respects. Suzy, Phil, and Sharon asked Abby to go to the diner after everything was done. They practically begged her to go. But Abby said she was tired and would just go home.

Abby hit a big box discount store on the way home, a store that kept a huge stock of Two-Dollar Dan on hand. Abby bought five containers.

Phil, Suzy, and Sharon, each called Abby at different times that evening. Between large glasses of Two-Dollar Dan, she assured each of them that she was fine and that she hadn't touched alcohol since the day she entered rehab.

Abby canceled plans with her mom to travel to Williamsburg, Virginia, later that week. She said she'd been feeling tired, like she had a bug, and didn't want to be a stick in the mud. By the end of the week, she had finished off seven containers of Two-Dollar Dan. For most adults, a moderate level of alcohol use consists of up to two drinks per day for men and one drink per day for women. A single five-ounce glass of wine equals one drink. But Abby was drinking 64 ounces of wine per day, which meant she was putting away almost 13 drinks per day and 91 drinks per week!

After two weeks of this drinking pattern, interspersed with phone calls from her mother, the remaining members of her peer group, and a few close friends, Abby finally realized how far she'd fallen off the wagon.

Sobering Up...Again

Abby's insurance benefits had remained intact during her "leave of absence." Once again, she got in touch with the school district's HR department. A HR representative helped secure resources that guaranteed her a spot in a medical detoxification program. The coverage, however, did not provide any reimbursement for an in-patient rehabilitation program.

By mid-July, Abby was sober again and had to figure out

how she could stay that way. But with the new school year on the horizon, the district needed to know by August 21st whether she would be starting the school year at Central. If she was not ready, the district would need to appoint a substitute until January 1st and keep Abby on leave until the end of winter vacation.

Abby didn't want to return to the AA meetings that followed her first rehab experience, and she wanted to earn a living. Given the deadline, she knew she needed help fast to get her life back on track. But she knew the deck might be stacked against her. For instance, she'd heard that people who have supportive spouses had a better chance of full recovery.

"Scratch that," she thought. "Thanks a lot, Steve."

And she knew of statistics saying that it takes between five and seven times for the average alcoholic to get sober. If she followed that pattern, she figured she would be kicked out of every school within a ten-state radius.

Abby decided to go back to her HR department and investigate resources that could provide her with the name of an in-network general practitioner who had experience in treating alcoholism.

A Good Candidate for Acamprosate

When Abby first met Dr. Gil Morris, he gave her a complete physical. He found that she had high blood pressure, high cholesterol, and fatty liver (a buildup of fat cells in the liver). He also administered the Alcohol Use Disorders Identification Test (AUDIT) to determine the extent of her alcohol dependence.

Luckily, Abby had remained sober since leaving the detox clinic. If she hadn't been sober, Dr. Morris explained that he would have had to negotiate a drinking goal with her before considering which medication could aid her battle. Her current sobriety meant that Dr. Morris could start her on a course of the drug acamprosate. Dr. Morris also found out that Abby was deficient in essential B vitamins, especially thiamin, and had low levels of chromium magnesium and selenium.

The Science of Acamprosate

Acamprosate, which also goes by the brand name Campral, was first legalized in France in 1989. It gained the (FDA) approval in the U.S. in 2004. By 2001, the effectiveness of acamprosate had already been evaluated via 16 controlled clinical trials in 11 European countries involving more than 4,500 alcohol-dependent outpatients. And by 2001, more than 1.4 million alcohol-dependent patients had been treated with the drug.

Acamprosate is commonly referred to as an anti-craving medication, but it may qualify more as a relapse-prevention drug.

People who try to recover from alcoholism often experience Post-acute Withdrawal Syndrome (PAWS). PAWS affects many aspects of recovery; it can interfere with a person's ability to keep a job or interact with family and friends. Its symptoms occur in 75 percent of people recovering from long-term alcohol use. Symptoms can include mood swings, problems thinking, and difficulty forming new memories.

PAWS may be partially due to adaptations in the central nervous system that occur as a result of growing tolerance, disturbances in neurotransmitters, and the resulting expectation of more activity (hyperexcitability) in nerve cells and brain systems. Neurotransmitters relay, amplify, and modulate signals between nerve cells (neurons) and other cells. PAWS symptoms may occur because the brain's ability to react to stress has been weakened by long-term alcohol abuse.

During recovery, especially early on, stressful situations arise, and symptoms of PAWS produce further distress. Therefore, alcoholics in withdrawal need to figure out ways to avoid or cope with triggers that can worsen PAWS. Acamprosate may be one way that helps alcoholics get over the hump and avoid those triggers.

The drug is composed primarily of acamprosate calcium, a synthetic compound with a chemical structure that resembles a naturally occurring amino acid. It appears to have a direct effect on reducing alcohol consumption, without residual effects on any functions or disorders in the central nervous system.

Although the exact action of acamprosate has not been determined, it appears to interfere with the brain processes that make alcoholics crave alcohol during withdrawal.

Acamprosate appears to restore normal glutamate activity in the brain. Glutamate is one of the brain's most common neurotransmitters, and is involved in almost all brain functions. The brain's glutamate system is a fast-signaling system that helps with information processing and long-term memory. This imbalance in glutamate occurs due to long-term alcohol abuse.

The glutamate system remains highly active and seeks out additional stimulation even after alcohol intake stops. That results in withdrawal symptoms. Nerve cells need to be "alcohol-free" for about one year or more to readjust properly.

Acamprosate is thought to stabilize that chemical imbalance by blocking glutamatergic *MGLUR2* receptors. Glutamatergic neurons control memory functions and synaptic plasticity - the ability of connections (synapses) between two nerve cells to adjust the strength accordingly. Synaptic plasticity also may play a role in a person's memory and learning ability. *N*-methyl-D-aspartate (NMDA) receptors are glutamate receptors; they seek out additional stimuli (they become "hyperexcited") as a result of chronic alcohol exposure.

Once glutamatergic NMDA receptors are blocked, it gives a chance for gamma-aminobutyric acid type A receptors (GABA-A) to be activated. GABA is the leading inhibitory neurotransmitter in the central nervous system (CNS); it quiets nerve impulses. GABA, which is directly responsible for regulating muscle tone, helps to regulate a nerve cell's ability to receive and respond to a stimulus throughout the CNS.

Success in Europe

In most European trials, differences in abstinence rates between study participants who took acamprosate versus those who took a placebo generally developed within the first 30 to 90 days of treatment. These rates were sustained for up to one year during treatment, and were maintained for as long as 12 months after treatment.

This was representative of studies that found acamprosate to be effective. The 2001 study was called *Acamprosate During and After Acute Alcohol Withdrawal: A Double-Blind Placebo-Controlled Study in Spain.*

In that study, acamprosate was introduced on the first day that patients began the process of detoxification. This allowed even patients who tended to drop out of studies midway to start the drug quickly this time. This strategy aided research; a body can only maintain a steady level of acamprosate beginning on the fifth day after the start of treatment. Being able to administer the drug quickly gave researchers a chance to measure optimal effects earlier, more than studies involving other drugs - which are usually measured a week or two after subjects begin alcohol withdrawal.

Results determined that the Cumulative Abstinence Duration (CAD, which is the length of time that abstinence was maintained) lasted about 93 days, 19 days longer for the acamprosate treatment group over the placebo treatment group. The stable recovery duration (the number of abstinent days between the last relapse and the end of the trial) was about 88 days, which was 16 days longer in the acamprosate treatment group than in the placebo group.

Acamprosate may have a greater success rate in Europe versus the United States due to societal disparities in the way long-term alcoholism is addressed. In Europe, many people who seek medical help with their alcoholism have been alcoholics longer and have more failed attempts at rehabilitation. Medically based or hospital-based treatment in Europe tends to be implemented after as many as five or six rehabilitation attempts. In the United States, the average person seeking medical help for alcoholism tends to visit a physician after two failed rehabilitation attempts and fewer years of steady drinking.

The long-term success of taking acamprosate has been

found to be most effective when combined with psychosocial component therapy, notably behavioral interventions focused on preventing relapse. Trials have not specified the exact components of such therapy, but like many other drug/behavioral therapy combinations, options range from simple interventions with physicians to full-blown support groups and/or extensive psychotherapy.

How Acamprosate Helps

Abby made a good candidate for acamprosate. Dr. Morris based his decision on two major factors:

Her family history; since Abby's father was at least partially alcohol dependent;

Her health conditions; Abby had high blood pressure, high cholesterol, and fatty liver. She, therefore, needed a medication that was not actively broken down (i.e., metabolized by the liver). Acamprosate is excreted by the kidneys unchanged.

Her recurrent post-withdrawal symptoms, which make her vulnerable to relapse, might also be diminished by acamprosate.

Almost everyone who drinks heavily has some form of fatty liver. Usually, there are no symptoms, but the liver may be enlarged and cause discomfort in the upper abdomen. The condition can improve after people stop drinking, but it could eventually lead to alcoholic hepatitis, an inflammation of the liver, and possibly cirrhosis. Cirrhosis occurs when normal liver tissue gets replaced with scar tissue.

Dr. Morris followed recommendations to introduce acamprosate using data she got from a publication in the American Family Physician - 2 tablets thrice a day (each tablet containing 333 mg of acamprosate). She advised Abby that she might have diarrhea or other side-effects of acamprosate, which could include dizziness, pruritus, and increased sexual desire. Infrequent adverse effects included insomnia, anxiety, depression, asthenia, nausea, vomiting, headache, drowsiness, dry mouth, paresthesias, and diaphoresis.

Dr. Morris also addressed the nutritional deficiencies using IV-vitamin substitution, which she started in the clinic, which after 2 sessions she switched to orally administered vitamins.

The doctor was also sensitized to Abby's special needs as a woman. Cleverly, she assigned her to sessions with an experienced female therapist who could combine specific aspects of CBT, stress-relief, and grief counseling. She also informed Abby that once she became more stable in treatment, they would spend more time examining her hormonal balance, which can either be a trigger or a consequence of alcohol use disorder. For many women, admitting to having an alcohol use disorder might be even more shameful than for most women, and there is usually a need for more engaged and direct psychological support. Dr. Morris knew that she had to keep a close eye on Abby to make sure that she did not develop a full-blown depressive illness, which would have required additional medicines. She was, however, comforted by the fact that should antidepressants become necessary, acamprosate would be a reasonable combination as it had few interactions with other medicines.

Few practices or addiction clinics cater specifically to women, and there is a large gap in the understanding of addressing all the needs of female patients with alcohol use disorder. Dr. Morris had, however, read an uplifting book called *"My way out"* by Roberta Jewell and Linda Garcia, M.D., in which the authors thanked a Prof. Dr. Bankole Johnson for their inspiration to find a women-focused innovative approach to curbing their alcohol addiction.

Coming Back

The administration of acamprosate, coupled with close monitoring and combined psychosocial support sessions from a psychologist, proved extremely effective for Abby. By mid-August, she hadn't taken a drink and felt no need to have one. She was able to meet the district's deadline for reporting that she would be able to start the school year back at Central.

She spent the last two weeks of August looking at lesson plans from past years to get back into the teaching groove. Already, Principal Riegel had called to say how eager he was to see her back in action. He also said the staff couldn't wait to see how she'd come dressed on the first day of school.

Abby felt her confidence coming back as the school approached. And despite not sleeping much the night before school started, she was rearing to go.

At 8:10 a.m., she made her way through lines of fourth, fifth, and sixth graders bellowing out sage offerings.

"Associate yourself with men of good quality if you esteem your own reputation. It is better to be alone than in bad company."

"Guard against the impostures of pretended patriotism."

"Has anyone seen my cherry tree?"

She was reciting the words of George Washington. And her outfit, complete with a bald wig, false teeth, and an accompanying ax, let everyone know that she was back to teach the kids of Central Middle School a thing or two.

Review

Alcohol Usage

For most adults, a moderate level of alcohol use consists of up to two drinks per day for men and one drink per day for women.

A single five-ounce glass of wine equals one drink.

It may take the average alcoholic seven times to get sober.

How Did Abby Get Help And Become A Good Candidate For Acamprosate?

Abby used her HR department to investigate family doctors in her insurance plan with experience in treating alcohol use disorder.

Her doctor gave her a complete physical and found that she had certain health conditions, which meant she needed medicine that was not metabolized by the liver:

High blood pressure.

High cholesterol.

Fatty liver.

Her doctor administered the Alcohol Use Disorders Identification Test (AUDIT) to determine the extent of her alcohol use disorder.

Her drinking patterns indicated a severe alcohol problem and difficulties stopping; however, these were interspersed with periods of abstinence she found hard to maintain.

Abby was drinking 64 ounces of wine per day, which equals about 13 drinks per day and 91 drinks per week.

Her family history indicated that Abby's father had alcohol use disorder

How Did Abby Get Help And Become A Good Candidate For Intravenous Vitamin Therapy?

Abby was deficient in B vitamins, especially thiamin. This would make her vulnerable to neurological diseases, including memory deficits. Thiamin is essential for normal neuronal functioning in the storage and retrieval of memories

Abby's vitamin deficiency had to be corrected quickly by intravenous infusion because a lack of B vitamins impairs the Kreb's cycle, thereby increasing the risks of abnormal glucose metabolism, diabetic ketoacidosis, coma, and even death

Chromium, selenium, and magnesium are all essential for normal brain function and development.

For a further review, see the chapters on restoration in this volume.

How Does Acamprosate Work?

Acamprosate also goes by the brand name Campral.

It was first legalized in France in 1989 and gained FDA approval in the U.S. in 2004.

It is commonly referred to as an anti-craving medication, but it may act more on relapse prevention. It may have a greater success rate in Europe versus the United States due to differences in the way long-term alcoholism is addressed.

It helps provide an opportunity to quiet nerve impulses.

The body can only maintain steady levels of acamprosate beginning on the fifth day after the start of treatment.

Long-term success rates of acamprosate have been found

to be most effective when combined with therapy focused on preventing relapse.

Therapy options can range from simple interventions with physicians to full-blown support groups and/or extensive psychotherapy.

Treatment And Follow-Up

Abby had regular weekly appointments with her doctor and psychologist for the first three months, and then this was switched to monthly visits for a following 6 months

Abby was reminded of alcohol's dangers by her doctor during regular visits.

Her blood work was analyzed regularly, and her doctor paid attention to her nutritional and hormonal needs.

Acamprosate helped Abby maintain sobriety and enabled her to return to her chosen occupation.

Stimulant Use Disorder:

Some myths...Some answers

Stimulants are drugs that have psychoactive properties. Unlike alcohol, which is usually only taken by mouth, stimulants can be smoked, snorted, injected, chewed, brewed in a drink, or taken as a pill. Synthetic stimulants are manufactured and have gained popularity because they are usually designed to produce heightened effects rapidly, and they are profitable to drug traffickers because they are typically easy to make - barely requiring more than a cursory knowledge of high school chemistry. Most stimulants are illegal substances, and their manufacture, distribution, or sale can lead to criminal prosecution and other penalties.

Up to 200 million Americans have used some type of stimulant in the past year. The most common stimulants include caffeine, nicotine, cocaine, methamphetamine, amphetamines and its analogies, electronic cigarettes, diet pills, plant stimulants, energy drinks, and varieties of bath salts. The following description of the actions of stimulants focuses on what is typically seen with cocaine, methamphetamine, and amphetamine analogs.

Stimulants have a powerful effect on brain function, where they generally produce alertness and increase vigilance. Even though these effects are desired among stimulant users, focused neuropsychological assessments typically do not report much in the way of improved executive functioning, and most of the performance gains are motoric. Other short-term effects of stimulants are to suppress appetite, elevate blood pressure, temperature, respiration, and heart rate. Sudden death from the use of stimulants usually results from cardiac arrest due to arrhythmias, myocardial infarction, and cerebrovascular ischemic or hemorrhagic stroke. Repeated stimulant use usually leads to addictive or neuropsychiatric disease. Upon initiation of stimulant use, users typically describe getting a "rush"; however, as the addiction deepens, users mostly report taking more stimulants to avoid the subsequent "crash" or depression as blood levels fall.

In women, the use of stimulants can lead to poor obstetric outcomes and harm to the developing fetus. There is an increased risk of preeclampsia, spontaneous abortion, and abruptio placentae, which can lead to the death of both mother and fetus. The babies of female stimulant users tend to be of low birth weight, small head circumference, and are at risk from cerebral infraction (i.e., a stroke). These babies tend to be very fussy, feed poorly, sleep irregularly, can develop tremors, and can be described as "jittery" babies that are hard to console. This severely disrupts early mother-baby bonding, which is critical for the normal healthy development of the baby.

Recreational use

As with alcohol, there are many myths pertaining the use of stimulants. One of these myths pertains to the supposition that recreational stimulant use does not lead to addiction. Recreational users use stimulants to alter their perceived mental state, and natural stimulants with psychedelic properties, like ayahuasca, are used to induce frank hallucinatory states on a voyage of apparent self-discovery. Ayahuasca is derived from the plant, Banisteriopsis cape, and it contains a large amount of monoamine oxidase inhibitors, which prevent the breakdown of monoamines. Ayahuasca is dangerous to use in the presence of tyramine, as this can provoke a hypertensive crisis and death. Other and more typical recreational uses of stimulants involve their use at parties, sporadic events, pill-popping in schools, or their use to control appetite and weight.

Irrespective of its nature of use, repeated use of stimulants can lead to addiction. The number of exposures is the determining factor in the development of addiction. The more you use stimulants, the greater the likelihood of developing an addiction.

Different strokes for different folk

Illicit stimulant users tend to make the choice of the agent between two main classes of drug - cocaine, and methamphetamine. The important difference is that whilst cocaine's effects peak rapidly (in minutes), those of methamphetamine can be sustained for several hours. Smoked methamphetamine's effects peak rapidly and decline slowly because of the greater length of time it takes for the body to break it down. This results in different drug-seeking patterns for users of cocaine and methamphetamine. For instance, cocaine users need to seek administration more frequently and go through more cycles of drug withdrawal compared to methamphetamine users. This phenomenon has led some clinicians to try and substitute cocaine for amphetamine analogs, but the results of these studies have been unconvincing as a viable treatment option.

Route of administration

The route by which a stimulant is taken into the body can affect its dangerousness. Intravenous administration (i.e., injecting directly into the bloodstream) is more dangerous than intranasal or oral administration because the effects are almost immediate. Intravenous use has further dangers associated with its administration such as the impurity of agents with which they are mixed. Also, the risk of sharing unsterilized needles and paraphernalia can increase the risk of local infections such as wound infections abscesses, and thrombophlebitis (inflamed blood vessels) and general infections like HIV, hepatitis, tuberculosis, lung infections including pneumonia (bacterial or viral), and renal infarction (damaged blood supply to the kidneys). Adulterants that are used, for example, to be mixed with cocaine, increase its "street" weight to maximize the profits of the drug dealer. Cocaine is typically mixed with lactose, mannitol, quinine, or glucose in proportion to mostly preserve its original taste

Inhalation is usually perceived by the user as the quickest way to ingest a stimulant, and evidence for that is borne by the popularity of "crack" cocaine and "ice" methamphetamine.

Nasal insufflation can have local consequences such as sinusitis, loss of smell, nasal congestion, reduced size of the nasal mucosa, difficulty with swallowing, and production of black sputum.

It's not easy to quit stimulants

There is ample folklore that it is easy to quit stimulant use, especially cocaine. Some would say that they have been life-long "chippers" using only at parties or specific events, and in between those times, they "can take it or leave it". Usually, a detailed history of stimulant use tends to elaborate on the true picture, and it is usual to discover that the reported sporadic use is several times a week and has been escalating over time. This is because, compared with alcohol, stimulants are more addictive as they have greater effects of stimulating the reward circuitry of the brain. Indeed, whilst alcohol is moderately addictive, most stimulants can be hundreds of times more reinforcing. Stimulants are more addictive than natural reinforcers, such as food and sex. In animal laboratories, it is easy to show that animals will ignore food and water to administer themselves more and more stimulants even up to the point of death if allowed. In humans, it is very much the same way as the reward circuitry is hijacked by the stimulant use such that it becomes the single over-riding objective for the individual. This sets up a dangerous spiral of deepening and dangerous stimulant use. In lectures, it is straightforward to teach college graduates this fact by asking them how easy it would be to give up sex? Then, ask them to consider doing so if it were up to a hundred times more rewarding? In the addiction world, it is relatively well known that it can be harder to get a smoker to quit using cigarettes compared with another individual to give up alcohol. The only difficulty with teaching this scenario is that up to 70 percent of individuals with alcohol use disorder also smoke, and that can complicate their recovery. An interesting experimental approach towards helping an individual reduce or stop stimulant use is to strengthen their executive functioning through a process called Trans Magnetic Stimulation (TMS). TMS is a noninvasive form of brain stimulation that applies powerful magnetic fields to specific regions of the brain. While it is not exactly clear how this technology works, individuals who receive this treatment sometimes report being able to forget or ignore the drive to use more stimulants.

Is there a role for talk therapy?

Several modalities of psychosocial treatment have been tried to help individuals with substance use disorder attain a drug-free status. Unfortunately, we seem to know a lot more about what does not work as opposed to what might work. For example, there is little evidence that intensive psychotherapy is beneficial, and the data on the utility of self-help groups is even thinner. Cognitive-Behavioral Treatment (CBT) has been shown to work for some individuals. CBT teaches the stimulant user skills to avoid high-risk situations where he or she may crave or desire to use more stimulants. An important aspect of engaging the stimulant user in treatment is a process called Motivational Interviewing (MI), which helps the individual to lay out the pros and cons of continued drug use and reinforce positive adaptive change towards clinical improvement. Perhaps the most convincing behavioral treatment to date has been contingency management, whereby the stimulant user exchanges money for foregoing or delaying using the stimulant. It is thought that by extending this delayed discounting that the stimulant use behavior diminishes and eventually extinguishes.

Is there a role for medication or other medical intervention?

No medicine has yet been established as a treatment for stimulant use disorder. In particular, more than 80 different medicines have been tried by the investigators associated with the National Institute on Drug Abuse (NIDA) to find a medicine to treat cocaine use disorder. One method that failed spectacularly was the use of medicines called dopamine antagonists. Stimulants have, in common, the effect to stimulate dopamine neurons in the reward circuitry of the corticomesolimbic area, which has been described above. The idea was to block this dopamine expression by simply using a blocker. The result in animals and somewhat in humans was that taking the dopamine blocker simply lead to greater desire and consumption of the stimulant to overcome the blockade. Attempts to give a less addictive stimulant to wean off a more powerful one also has been tried with limited success, and so has an approach to give a medicine that can act at times like direct mixed agonist/antagonists; again, with no success. One approach that has shown some early promise that was pioneered by the author of this book is the use of topiramate, which has complex actions as multiple receptors and principally as both an indirect stimulator/and inhibitor; however, this is still an experimental approach and more studies are needed to validate this early finding. This author plans to implement a precision medicine approach to identify potential responders to treatment better.

There is growing evidence that TMS may reduce the craving for cocaine. This is a promising experimental procedure that could be applied generally in clinical practice if larger studies prove to be effective. Some technical kinks still need to be ironed out to determine the exact protocols that would lead to the most effective clinical response. This author believes that one way in which this research could be embellished would be to compare genetic expressions between responders and non-responders and use this approach to identify target genes and genotypes for a precision medicine approach to treatment.

Comorbidity

An important aspect of the treatment of an individual with stimulant use disorder is comorbidity. The myth of the regular stimulant user with no neuropsychiatric consequences is just that - a myth. Stimulant use can itself be a symptom of an underlying serious psychiatric disease, notably bipolar disorder, a condition in which the afflicted individual can experience wild mood swings from frank mania to the depths of depression. Bipolar disorder is the most heritable of neuropsychiatric diseases. Stimulant users also appear to be prone to depression and suicidality, which must be specifically inquired about when an individual presents for treatment.

Additionally, stimulant users often have added substance use disorders, particularly alcohol.

Synthetic stimulants can have untoward and unexpected effects, depending on how they are blended or laced with other chemicals or impurities. There is a myth that synthetic stimulants may be safer than naturally occurring stimulants like cocaine, but the opposite is the more likely scenario. Synthetic stimulants have been associated with altered personality, mood swings, aggression, and, at times, extreme violence due to the rapid dissociation of the individual from the ability to make rational executive decisions.

Do stimulants have any uses?

Stimulants have a long history of being used to treat medical conditions, and a significant amount of their misuse originates from diversion. Notably, stimulants such as Ritalin and Adderall have been used to treat attention deficit hyperactivity disorder (ADHD). Modafinil has been used to treat a sleep condition called narcolepsy, and weaker amphetamine analogs have been used to control obesity. All these medicines rely on their ability to increase levels of monoamines (norepinephrine, epinephrine, serotonin, and/or dopamine) in the blood, and differ in the proportion by which they elevate each of them.

Where do we go from here?

Educating the stimulant user about the short- and long-term consequences of use is key to making progress in treatment. A physical examination and detailed health inquiry are essential. Women of childbearing age will need a specialist gynecological/obstetric evaluation. If the female stimulant user has any children, an evaluation of their physical and mental health should be considered.

Key to the addiction management of an individual with stimulant use disorder is the personalization of the approach, which starts from the history taking. A MI approach is, perhaps, optimal to initially building rapport and confidence in the treatment provider. Care should be taken in the next steps to establish a foundation for further psychosocial treatment, which is best undertaken to target the critical provoking or perpetuating factors associated with the stimulant use.

Clearly, the "silver bullet" and "one size fits all" approach to finding an effective medical approach to treating substance use disorder has not been successful and needs to be abandoned for more precision-based approaches to treatment. On an individual patient level, it may have ethical merit, having carefully explained the pros and cons to the individual with substance use disorder. Evidently, those who choose to participate in this quasi-experiment will help to develop these approaches, and at a micro-level, by individualizing the treatment to find what works, one patient at a time helps to build the armamentarium of approaches that might work for many others.

* * *

Signature Reflection: The Star Teacher

Abby holds a classroom together while her private world quietly unravels. The story honors the particular danger of "functional" suffering - the kind that still grades papers, still smiles, still bleeds in silence. Early sobriety is not just bravery; it is physiology - stabilized, supported, made possible.

If you remember one thing: asking for help is a form of professionalism.

- The dragon's disguise: competence that hides pain - and a bottle that becomes a private anesthetic.
- The turning point: turning toward care (support + medication + follow-up) instead of muscling through alone.
- A practice to try: choose one person to tell the truth to. One sentence. No speech. Just honesty.

Clinical lens: after stopping alcohol, the brain's excitatory systems can rebound. Medications like acamprosate, paired with support, can make the early weeks more tolerable and reduce relapse risk.

The Wild Child

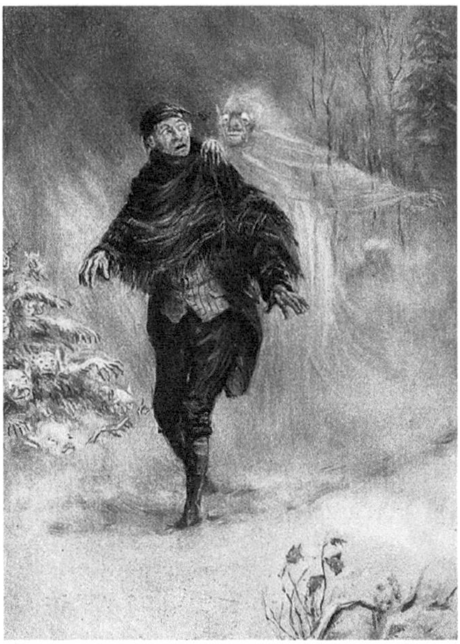

The image above is: Illustration by Frederick Simpson Coburn.

Frederick Simpson Coburn's illustration - *What fearful shapes and shadows beset his path amidst the dim and ghastly glare of a snowy night* - appeared in a British Library publication and was later discussed in Richard Millington's "Wild Heart Turning White" (The Public Domain Review), written in reflection on poet Georg Trakl's turbulent life and death.

The image turns snow into something ominous - light made hostile. In Millington's commentary, the motif evokes cocaine's double promise: exhilaration at first, self-destruction in the end. It foreshadows Jeremy's story here: brilliance chased by consequences, a man fleeing an inner pursuer he can't outpace.

This story begins with a physician's alarm bell and widens into a patient's. It is a reminder that treatment is not only what we prescribe - it is what we model: urgency when the body says "stop," and humility when the mind says "I can handle it alone."

He'd lived with migraines for years, but this one was different. The familiar flicker at the edge of vision arrived like lightning strikes - brief, violent flashes that made the room seem to strobe. Then came the darker symptom: flecks, like charcoal suspended in air, drifting across his visual field.

He had always loved Lewis Carroll's description of Alice's distortions - how a migraine can make the world bend. But this didn't feel like whimsy. Those black specks weren't in front of him; they were inside his eye. Retinal detachment? An ophthalmic migraine? His mind ran the differential as fear sharpened it: how quickly could vision be lost, and how permanent could the damage become?

Harrow's Field Note: When the Body Rings the Alarm

John woke with a headache that felt like a warning.

He had always suffered from migraines, but this one was different. Not only was he getting the usual flashing lights in his peripheral vision, but this time, they were like lightning strikes. It was as if the whole room was lighting up, but this was no *aurora borealis*. There was no beauty or mystery to this, and, adding to it, were these flecks of dark charcoal-like particles floating in front of his visual field.

John had enjoyed the stories of Lewis Carroll, and his vivid description (or better yet, hallucination) of *Alice in Wonderland* that had seemingly been invoked by a migraine headache. He knew that this was potentially more serious and that the charcoal-like particles were not in front of him, but inside of his eye. Could these be parts of his retina separating from the back of his eye? Soon, he could lose his vision, and if not repaired, the damage could be permanent. John knew that this was either an impending or partial retinal detachment or at best, an ophthalmic migraine, or worse. And how could it really be worse?

The Meeting

John recalled one of his first patients who had presented with an ophthalmic headache. However, what he recalled about this strange man was much more than his florid descriptions about his headache; it was his wild character. Jeremy and John had become friends but only spoke on New Year's Eve to sing Auld Lang Syne together. Jeremy knew all the words of this Robert Burns poem, which was composed in 1788. Jeremy was born on the west side of Glasgow to a family of doctors, who had, remarkably, brought seven other siblings to life. He always finished the song with a warning: 'It's always later than you think.'

As the years had passed, this warning haunted John, as he could not permit himself to think of endings. There was simply too much to do. But he knew that nature would not allow a vacuum and as one passed on, those about to step in his or her place would all take their places behind in the line.

Jeremy, given his upbringing on the west side of Glasgow, could not be described as shy. He had a lanky frame, nicely manicured mustache, and paid considerable attention to the shoes he wore. He had made his money, indeed quite a fortune, in the City of London as a Forex trader. Jeremy was, simply, brilliant at any kind of mental arithmetic and often mocked his fellow traders who had to resort to mere computers. As he would say, when asked about his profession:

"I sell money to people for as much as I can get, and then buy it back for a steal because they usually buy more than they need. Selling money is like selling fresh fruit; buy too much, and it has to be given or thrown away before it completely rots."

It was, therefore, fairly apt that Jeremy was usually fond of recounting that the shoes worn by a man were the true eye into his soul, and it was better to wear tatty clothes rather than unkempt boots. Jeremy's favorite shoes were a pair of cowboy boots that he had been given by a Texan oilman, who had insisted that he fly to San Antonio to get his lasts and fittings done. That way, he could always order another pair of boots that he fancied simply by calling the store, confident in the knowledge that they would fit perfectly upon arrival. Now, how many places in the world offered this kind of luxury anymore? His lasts would remain at Little's boots, in a climate-controlled room in San Antonio, for as long as this family business existed. Little's boots specialty was exotic, unvarnished leathers, and Jeremy had settled for a pair of half-calf high Ostrich boots that could be worn on any occasion. Jeremy swore, as most do, that these were truly the best boots in the world. To anyone who met him cursorily, Jeremy was the ultimate gentleman, but that impression only lasted a few minutes if he took you out into the town.

A Happy New Year?

John had decided for some reason to make the New Year's call a little early. It was about 9 pm in Scotland when Jeremy received the call.

"Happy New Year in advance," belted John as soon as the phone was answered.

There came a long pause, and then a response by an unfamiliar voice.

"Jeremy is that you?" asked John.

"Of course. Yes," Jeremy replied.

"Well, why do you sound so strange? It's as though you were at the bottom of a well, and talking through your nose," followed John.

There was another long pause, followed by what sounded like a yawn. John checked his watch and the setting for the dual time phase. Surely, it was still just 9 pm in Scotland. And so, it was.

"Have you been feeling unwell, or did the celebrations start early for you?" asked John. Being met with silence, he continued. "Over here, the fireworks start at about 6 pm. I call these folk *plonkers* with not much else to do. And in the middle of Miami, it's like party central all day long at New Year's."

Jeremy took his time in answering. "It's been quite a year, and I am very happy to see the end of it. Busy as hell, with not so much as a minute to myself. And then mom died, and I had to put dad in a home - absolutely horrible business. The firm's been doing so well though that they brought in these newbies from big universities. You would expect that with all their high falutin education, someone would have taught them how to think. Instead, they simply keep pushing buttons on their computer, hoping that the right output will occur, as if by magic."

John did not interrupt. It seemed like Jeremy needed someone to vent to, and, after all, it was only once a year.

Jeremy went on. "I have a friend in Miami, other than you, who got into a spot of bother lately. He was caught snorting cocaine at work, and his whole world came crashing down the day his employment was terminated. Terrible business. May I refer him to you in the New Year?"

"Certainly," replied John. "You know my number. Just have him give me a call to set up an appointment. Better still, it seems like I have Jan. 4th completely open. I can dedicate that day to him. It's usually our first day back at work, and we do not typically schedule any patients, but since it's a friend of yours, we'll make an exception."

"That would be super," Jeremy answered. "And, by the way, have a happy New Year."

John had thought no more of the conversation when he arrived at work on the scheduled day. All the staff had turned up to the clinic and descended first into a quiet chatter, and then noisy laughter, and finally, the wild shouting was just mayhem. Everyone was in the best of moods.

"John, someone is waiting for you at reception, and he refuses to give his name. He says you would wish to see him," said the front door assistant who had called John on his telephone.

On almost any other day, John would have insisted on knowing who it was, but then he remembered that Jeremy's friend might be coming through for a visit. John opened the connecting door to the clinic, which was about 50 feet from the front entrance. The figure in the distance looked somewhat familiar, and as he got closer, more familiar indeed. It was Jeremy!

"What in blue blazes are you here for Jeremy? Of course, I'm delighted to see you. Did you bring your friend with you?" John asked quizzically.

Jeremy looked left, then right, then at his feet. "Just me," he said in a barely audible voice.

Shame vs. Despair

John knew of the shame that can infect many an addict. If John was a top heart surgeon and a friend needed heart surgery, guess who would be called first? You could apply this logic to almost any kind of medical disease except for disorders of the mind, or worse, diseases that some perceive the afflicted brought upon themselves by being careless, stupid, or reckless...or, all at the very same time. For those people, having an addiction was an emblem of failure, and a demonstration of a lack of self-control and personal willpower to stay on the straight and narrow path of decency. Intelligent and successful people should not end up being addicts because they were meant to know when to stop before it became so serious.

John had found himself in florid debates with people who thought this way. It was not enough for him to explain to them that the circuits in the brain that were associated with reinforcing important behaviors that led to a positive life were the very same ones that had been highjacked by the disease. He also found it no good explaining that after over a hundred years of extensive psychological research, no one had, as yet, defined scientifically an “addictive personality,” and that this concept was enshrined in fiction to demonize the addict. He had given up on these arguments, likening them to a living person describing what it must be like to be dead to someone who was, in fact dead, and providing contradictory information. Arguments in different planes of thought never really converged to reason or the satisfaction of most.

John was not ashamed of his friend. Indeed, he was proud of him!

“Team,” he announced, “this is Jeremy, an old friend of mine. He is here today to start a new path to recovery, as we have helped so many to do. And he’s here all the way from Scotland.”

The team broke up their small gathering and took to their stations. John explained to Jeremy that since they were good friends, it would be better if he saw Dr. Nimrod, but that John would remain present to provide assistance and guidance as needed.

The Fight

Dr. Nimrod ushered Jeremy into his cozy office and started by asking him, "What is it that you do not like about your behavior, and how can we help? Please start from anywhere you wish to."

For the first time that morning, Jeremy looked up and started to talk.

"I really do not like anything about myself anymore. I am not the man I used to be. A few weeks ago, I was at a quaint little pub on the west side of Glasgow, nursing a single malt with my girlfriend, Elena, and her brother Sam. It was such a lovely pub, and the people who come here have been doing so for years! Up till then, my life had been one of moderation while at home, but once I go through my front door, the partying really started. I had not known Elena long, but our relationship had long periods of separation. I knew she dated other men, but I did not know the true extent of it. At one point, when we were talking about the demise of Scottish football, Elena's face suddenly glowed red hot as she started to cry. She screamed; 'I was raped last week, why hasn't anyone noticed?'

"I went to throw my arms around her to comfort her, but she recoiled. I was shocked when she pointed at me. 'It was you!' she exclaimed. It was if I had fallen off a boat and could not breathe in the water, as the other nearby guests turned around. Elena did not look that drunk, and I tried to make sense of things, but before I could say anything, Sam had hit me in the mouth without a moment's hesitation. The last thing

I remembered about that night was waking up in the hospital, answering the questions of the local constabulary.

"'You're very lucky to be alive,' the policeman had said. 'Although, it might have been better if we had left you for dead from what we heard. You took quite some beating to the head,'" Jeremy continued narrating.

"It turned out that Elena had got her story all mixed up, and the man who had assaulted her was a passing acquaintance she picked up whilst working as a part-time escort to get some "pocket money" to boost her wages as a struggling architect. All of this had happened to her in an alcohol-infused haze, and now it was too late to find the culprit or press charges. The crux of the matter was that the way I was leading my life, I could not remember anything, and it might very well have been me who had assaulted Elena. You see, trouble had started a few months earlier. Sam was not just Elena's brother; he had also been bringing me the "white stuff" to pick up my mood."

"You mean cocaine?" asked Dr. Nimrod.

Jeremy nodded.

"I would do a few lines at home late in the evening and then try my hand at online gambling. After all, I should have been good at gambling; I did it every day for real with billions of other people's money. I did not lose much at the beginning, but as my losses grew, I started to "chase" them. Just one more round would set me right, I thought. But it never did. The more money I lost, the more I gambled. I have lost almost everything I have, but I can tell you now, if you put cocaine in front of me now, I would snort it. It's getting harder, though, because my nasal septum has collapsed, and I have had to resort to "popping" the cocaine through my skin at times. I just cannot stop!"

Jeremy rolled up his sleeves and showed Dr. Nimrod the deep scars and abrasions on his arms.

The Future of the Science of Addiction, Now?

Dr. Nimrod was experienced enough to let Jeremy tell his story. He remembered what his teachers had banged into his head - the patient will tell you the diagnosis!

"The first thing we have to do is to see how badly damaged your brain is. We will do this over several tests. First, we will have you take a neurocognitive exam," he said.

"Like an IQ test?" asked Jeremy.

"Well, the test can tell us your IQ, but more importantly, it will tell us how efficiently different parts of your brain are working. Then we combine that knowledge with a special scan of your brain called an MRI (Magnetic Resonance Image), which tells us whether different parts of your brain are working properly. An MRI does this by generating a magnetic field, magnetic field gradients, and radio waves to take pictures of the metabolism of different parts of the brain. It is not like an x-ray as it does not contain ionizing radiation. In your case, we need to do a special MRI with diffusion tensor imaging, because when you were knocked out, it is possible that sensitive parts of your brain might have been damaged. Certain types of brain damage could also make it harder for you to be able to give up cocaine. We also need to get your clinical notes from the Royal Infirmary in Glasgow, where you were taken after you were rendered unconscious. It's a great hospital, John can attest to this as he did some of his training there."

"Is that all?" asked Jeremy.

"Not quite," replied Dr. Nimrod. He continued. "We will be running additional tests for the rest of the week, including your blood work, to check your complete physical status; genetic profile, to determine which medicines we can give you and in what amount; and further psychological assessments of your mood and daily living capacity. Don't worry, our job is to get you in tip-top shape. After all the examination results are in, all our doctors and health care providers will meet to determine your treatment plan. We will also have some "special" help, and I guess you will like this, from computer algorithms that will "learn" your response to our treatments, so if we do not get it spot-on the first time, we certainly shall in subsequent visits."

Jeremy's interest was now piqued. "All this sounds like science fiction; I never knew a place like this existed," he said.

"Well, we call it the future of the science of addiction now, and our motto is *beyond science...and beyond borders.TM* We incorporate the very latest of what is known into our delivery system," said Dr. Nimrod proudly.

Jeremy found the first four days to be a blur of testing, and even more testing, before finally, the day arrived for him to meet again with the team. Dr. Nimrod, sitting at the top of the table, led the meeting. Jeremy watched and listened as each expert he had seen delivered their views regarding his condition in a way that built a full picture of who he was at a personal level. He was the center of attention, and he knew that their treatment recommendation would not be a cookie-cutter one size fits all approach, but a regimen that was tailored specifically for him.

The Diagnoses

Finally, Dr. Nimrod began his summary.

"Jeremy, let's start with the obvious and what you know and do not like about yourself. You have both a cocaine use disorder and a gambling disorder. We followed up with your history at Royal infirmary when you had a head injury. You seem to have been lucky - your Glasgow Coma scale score was 14, indicating that any injury you suffered to the brain was mild. Although you do not meet diagnostic criteria for major depression, your mood is certainly gloomy. Concerning your cognitive performance, there is evidence of hesitation and approximations on your part. In very bright people like yourself, when your brain cannot work out the right answer from memory or being able to calculate, you start to "guess". We noted that your heart is beating too fast (this is called tachycardia) and occasionally skips a beat. Although this is not dangerous, we have to be careful to monitor it properly. For instance, a common mistake some doctors make is to prescribe a drug called a beta-blocker that reduces norepinephrine levels to slow the heart down. But we do not do that because beta-blockers can cause the small blood vessels of the heart to shut down. Because cocaine also can shut down the very same blood vessels, some cocaine users can develop a heart attack and die from this simple mistake."

Jeremy gasped audibly and coughed nervously.

Dr. Nimrod continued with his analysis. "We also noticed from your blood work that you have not been looking after yourself or eating properly. In particular, you are low on vitamins B, D, and E. Now, these are not dangerously low, but they still need to be corrected to prevent future health problems. And, let's not forget about those headaches you used to have all those years ago. I am glad they have lessened in intensity."

Jeremy looked frightened, and Dr. Nimrod paused for Jeremy's emotions to catch up with what he was hearing. Like a schoolboy, the patient put his hand up before starting to speak.

"It seems like I'm going to be with you for years. I simply cannot take any more bad news."

Dr. John looked at his friend and smiled. His kind eyes said it all before he could speak the words.

"Jeremy, you will only be with us for about another month until we get you stabilized. You can stay in the hotel above our offices so it would be easy for you to come down and see us every time we need to see you. Or, we can simply come up to your room to administer some of the treatments, if it is easier for you to feel more comfortable there. Your time with us will go by very quickly. You'll see."

Jeremy looked re-assured and put his hands down.

Jeremy Finally Gets Help

Dr. Nimrod changed his posture and was now looking directly at Jeremy. He started to speak again.

"The good news is that we have everything here to help you, but it is going to be a good deal of work to cram into a month. We have had an extensive discussion with the team and have come up with a plan. We have decided to progress trying some highly personalized experimental treatments, with the goal of tackling many problems at once, rather than your having to undergo a multitude of procedures, or worse, leave here rattling with bottles of pills."

Jeremy gave a wry smile, appreciating somewhat Dr. Nimrod's approach to lightening the mood. But then, he jerked himself back into listening mode as the serious part was now coming up.

Signature Scene: The Weight of Experimental Hope

John listened as Jeremy tried to joke his way past fear, and he felt the familiar pull in his own chest - the clinician's urge to reassure, the friend's urge to promise. Both urges were dangerous.

Experimental treatments live in a strange moral space. You can see the logic. You can cite the early data. You can explain mechanisms until the room feels safe again. But in the end, you are still asking a human being to step into uncertainty in exchange for a chance at relief.

John thought of his migraine that morning - the way the body can ring an alarm bell before the mind is ready to hear it. Jeremy's alarm was louder: cocaine, gambling, depression, a damaged heart. The dragon here had multiple heads, and every head had its own hunger.

He watched Jeremy's hands, the subtle tremor when the conversation grew too real. This was not a man who needed a speech. This was a man who needed options, honesty, and a plan concrete enough to hold when craving hit.

"Here is what we know," John began, choosing precision over comfort. "Here is what we don't know. Here is what we will measure, session by session. And here is what you get to decide." In that moment, hope did not feel like a slogan. It felt like informed consent - dignity returned to the person who had been losing control.

Transcranial Magnetic Stimulation (TMS)

Dr. Nimrod was now in full "doctor mode" as he started up again.

"To treat your cocaine use disorder, gambling, and depressed mood, we are going to try an experimental procedure called Trans-Magnetic Stimulation (TMS). TMS is still experimental for the treatment of cocaine use disorder, and the evidence for its utility in gambling disorder is anecdotal. TMS is a non-invasive form of brain stimulation. TMS works by applying strong magnetic fields to specific parts of the brain to enhance activity. Basically, some of the clinicians that initially started to use TMS for different conditions found that those who gambled seemed to lose their propensity to do so. There is evidence TMS can help with migraines, but we are not expecting that, since ophthalmic migraines, like you and John suffer from, seem pretty unresponsive to anything we can throw at it. The stress you have suffered as a result of your assault also might be helped by TMS. TMS usually has a few side-effects, the most common being headaches, but more serious consequences such as seizure have been described. Of course, we will provide you with a full information sheet pertaining to all the possible side effects. I want to stress that TMS is still considered experimental for most of the conditions you have (except, perhaps, depression), and you have a choice to refuse this treatment.

"For us to start TMS, you will need to give us your informed consent, knowing that it is experimental, and that data is still being collected pertaining to its efficacy and suitability for use in treating your medical conditions. We do, however, think this is a good initial plan, as it personalizes an approach to treating you directly for several considerable medical challenges - all at the same time whilst minimizing side-effects, and avoiding polypharmacy (i.e., the use of many medications to treat a single individual who has a multitude of symptoms). We are comfortable administering TMS to you because even though you suffered a head injury, your score on the Glasgow Coma scale was quite high, and the special Diffusion Tensor MRI did not show any micro-bleeds in the brain. Furthermore, our regular MRI scans during your TMS treatment will let us pick up any problems very early," the doctor finished.

Jeremy put his hand up like a shot and asked, "So, what brain areas will you be applying the TMS to, how do you know I got enough stimulation, and how many sessions do I need?"

Dr. Nimrod was quick to respond. "You are asking all the right questions, Jeremy. Before we start, we will test your eligibility for TMS by administering a safety screen (Rossi et al. 2011), and only if you qualify would we get you to sign the informed consent form. Once we are clear with all of that, we can choose from several different protocols. However, the one we favor the most is stimulation of a part of the brain called the dorsolateral prefrontal cortex (DLPFC). Because of our access to MRI, we will use that technology to navigate exactly where to place the coil, so this will be calibrated perfectly for you from the first session to the last. We will perform another check, which would be to dial in the intensity of stimulus until we can excite your motor cortex to elicit movement. That strength of stimulus is what we will use during the remainder of the TMS treatment sessions to excite the DLPFC. We will be careful to test our mapping by stimulating a "landmark" area such as the motor cortex. Our team will aim to get in at least 20 sessions over the next month, so we will have to see you daily. We will be absolutely as precise as possible."

Hyperbaric Oxygen Treatment

Dr. Nimrod was not finished.

"Jeremy, we also need to try to add some other treatments. We would like to have you undergo hyperbaric oxygen treatment. Even though your concussion was mild, such events in the brain disrupt normal blood flow and oxygenation. It would, therefore, be reasonable to propose that the symptoms of depression and the memory difficulties that you are having could imply that you remain at risk for post-concussion syndrome. Chronic cocaine use also reduces brain oxygenation, so the combination of both events has probably added up for you. Hyperbaric treatment increases oxygenation to the brain and heals these brain "wounds" by increasing the release of stem cells. These stem cells cause a phenomenon called angiogenesis (i.e., the formation of new capillaries) in the brain. Although there remains some controversy with hyperbaric oxygen treatment, there really is some very exciting and clever work being done by Dr. Shai Efrati's team in Israel (Boussi-Gross et al. 2013). We will pair your TMS and hyperbaric oxygen treatments on the same day to get you the maximum benefit."

Cognitive restructuring, relapse prevention, and exercise

Dr. Nimrod was now beginning to wrap up his long summary.

"Jeremy, we also need to get you into better psychological and physical shape. We will add a regimen of targeted cognitive restructuring to improve your memory with relapse prevention skills (to increase your ability to avoid high-risk situations for using cocaine and gambling). We have an absolutely brilliant neuropsychologist who can combine both to save time, and tailor what you need specifically for you. She will educate you about the dangers of needle use, which can cause hepatitis, HIV, and other infections. The vitamin deficiencies will be easy to cure by just providing you with a suitable set of vitamin infusions. Last, but perhaps not least, our physiotherapist has devised a set of 30-min aerobic exercises for you, which will not only improve your physical conditioning but also can improve brain oxygenation. In some studies, aerobic exercise has been shown to improve depression (Blumenthal et al. 2012), decrease brain aging, improve memory, and decrease stress (Ahlskog et al. 2011). And that's about it, Jeremy. Any questions?"

Jeremy did not know where to start. This was not his image of recovery from addiction and gambling. Nothing he had watched or read had prepared him for anything like this. So much applied science, all condensed into a precise package just for him. Jeremy decided that rather than ask his questions at this meeting, he would use his month at the clinic to educate himself and take his time to speak and learn from all the professionals on the team.

Saying goodbye

Jeremy was a very different man five weeks later as he bid goodbye to the clinical team who had arranged a schedule to follow up with him by videoconferencing, and trips back every month to calibrate and increase the precision of these treatments. He did have some cravings to use cocaine and gamble remaining, but these he could now ignore using his relapse prevention skills. Jeremy was no longer using cocaine or gambling.

Finding Elena

Still, there was unfinished business. On this trip back home, flying "across the pond" to Scotland, Jeremy knew he had to find Elena. None of her old numbers worked, and only by luck did he come across the number of a friend of hers. Jeremy and Elena agreed to meet a few weeks later. Elena had spent the past two months going to intensive crisis groups for women who had been the victim of a sexual assault and had alcohol and/or substance use disorders. For Elena, this active support group was all that she needed. She was not "brand new," but was coping, and had found a proper full-time job in her trained profession as an architect. Elena was on a journey that would take her many months, perhaps years, to get back to being able to trust anyone. Jeremy and Elena never met again after that brief reunion. The scars were simply too deep, and they both decided to leave their skeletons well buried, comfortable in the knowledge that they had at least forgiven each other for the past.

John gets help for his ophthalmic migraine

John had heard all the stories of "healing the healer", and decided to visit the Bascom Palmer Eye Institute at the University of Miami to investigate his visual disturbances and headaches. Like in his own field, this institute was the zenith in the USA for the treatment of eye diseases, and he enjoyed the elderly but uniquely clever doctor who looked after him. John was lucky, his retina had not detached, although he now had to learn to live with those occasional ophthalmic headaches. Quiet meditation, and listening to Johan Sebastian Bach's violin concerto no.1 in A minor recorded by Daniel Lozakovich, a musical genius, for Deutsche Grammophon or the violin solo no.2 in A minor recorded by DECCA and played by Hilary Hahn, another prodigious talent, always seemed to do the trick for him.

Simply put, their playing is what he imagined God's angels would sound like in heaven! Perhaps, one day there will be a cure for his peculiar migraine; but then, something would be missing. The luxury of time for himself, a greedy pleasure, and a commodity, which was now all too precious to delete from his "busy" schedule.

The journey continues...

For John, the journey continues each and every day, learning from his patients. Now, could that be the ultimate joy?

Review

Jeremy's case was quite complicated since he had significant comorbid disorder rather than just cocaine use disorder. This required an "out of the box" treatment approach, which was highly personalized towards him. Of course, with such a complex case, there were opportunities the treatment team considered but rejected. For instance, the team could have attempted to use topiramate to curb his cocaine addiction, which was another experimental approach pioneered by this author. As a first-line approach, that would, however, have locked the team into a plethora of add-on treatments. Basically, they tried to find a solution that addressed the bulk of his problems at the same time. Indeed, every modality of treatment chosen by the team was woven intimately to "heal" the brain and reduce oxidative, and inflammatory stresses to the brain. Concerning decision-making, the team took the approach to personalize his treatment as much as possible. Jeremy experienced remarkable success with this approach. All those who seek treatment are, however, different and so can their responses be. The programmed approach the team took left room for flexibility and alterations in the type and timing of the approach. Finally, the team took into consideration Jeremy's wishes, timeframe, and lifestyle to optimize their approach.

Introduction To Opioid Use Disorder -

Just A Few Useful Facts

The USA is in the grip of an opioid use disorder (now an epidemic), which is a leading cause of death. In 2018, 46,802 people died from a fatal overdose of opioids. Deaths from opioid overdose accounted for about two-thirds of all overdose deaths in the USA. The states with the highest overdose deaths were: West Virginia (51.5/100,000); Delaware (43.8/100,000); Maryland (37.2/100,000; Pennsylvania (36.1/100,000); Ohio (35.9/100,000), and New Hampshire (35.8/100,000).

Opioids consist of a range of substances that bind tightly to the opioid receptors in the brain to produce euphoria and pain relief. The primary medicinal use of opioids is for the relief of pain.

Notable among the class of opioid drugs are heroin, morphine, fentanyl, codeine, hydrocodone, and oxycodone. Because of the explosion in the prescription of opioids for pain relief, the passing or sale of the prescribed medicine is the common method of diversion.

Over 2 million people in the USA have a substance use disorder caused by the over-prescription of opioid pain medicines. However, in 2016, it was estimated that only about 17.6% of them received specialist treatment. Importantly, the opioid crisis has caused a dramatic rise of infants being born to mothers' dependent on opioids, children with neonatal abstinence syndrome when they are born, and increased the spread of infectious diseases, including hepatitis and HIV.

Opioid use disorder (OUD) is frequently associated with alcohol use disorder (AUD), which corresponds to an increased risk of mortality, morbidity, and psychosocial impairment. AUD is also associated with an enhanced risk of fatal overdose in OUD, along with an increase in hepatotoxicity in hepatitis-positive individuals, and accelerated liver cirrhosis. AUD among individuals with OUD is also a strong predictor of negative outcomes, with lowered compliance to treatment, impaired social functioning, and quality of life.

Prevention and treatment services are not well utilized, and even where they exist, are organized poorly (The author of this volume led the clinical component and was involved intimately with the Maryland Governor's Heroin and Opioid Emergency Task Force 2015). The poor outcomes of present services can be enhanced by: significantly increasing access to treatment, especially in office-based settings; disseminating information concerning the use of medicines to reverse the sedative effects of opioids, increasing public health surveillance; promoting cutting-edge research, and ensuring that best practices in pain management are adhered to and encouraged.

Most individuals with OUD who undergo detoxification and, subsequently, proceed with following a complete abstinence program, irrespective of the level of psychosocial support provided, will relapse, and this increases the risk of fatal overdose. Without medication-assisted treatment (MAT), the management of those with an opioid disorder who have recently been detoxified is likely to result in failure.

Whilst the Food and Drug Administration recently approved lofexidine (which activates the adrenergic-2 receptor) in 2018, the first non-opioid medicine for the treatment of OUD, the mainstay of MAT for the treatment of OUD are those that have a direct effect on the opioid system and its receptors.

Methadone is a synthetic opioid agonist (i.e., it excites opioid receptors), and its primary use is to decrease withdrawal symptoms. By reducing withdrawal symptoms, negative emotions that can give rise to cravings are diminished. Methadone's activation of opioid receptors is slow and, at the usual prescribed dose, does not induce euphoria in individuals with OUD. Methadone is prescribed by specialist addiction centers and has been in use since 1947.

Buprenorphine excites the opioid receptors but not as strongly as other opiates. It is, therefore, considered to be a partial agonist at opioid receptors. Buprenorphine can reduce cravings and withdrawal symptoms among those with OUD and has similar efficacy to methadone. Buprenorphine was approved by the FDA in 2002, primarily to be used in office-based practices, which are widespread, instead of the usual specialized treatment services. The Comprehensive Addiction Recovery Act (CARA) of 2016 expanded the use of buprenorphine for prescription by nurse practitioners and physician assistants. Buprenorphine can be taken in several different ways, such as, as a sublingual (under the tongue) preparation, a 6-month subdermal implant, and as a monthly injection.

In contrast to opioid agonist treatment, naltrexone is an opioid antagonist (i.e., it blocks opioid receptors) and prevents the actions of other opioids. Among individuals with OUD, naltrexone will be associated with withdrawal symptoms, and its use is optimized for aiding those who are already abstinent to remain in that condition. The injectable form of naltrexone, naloxone, is used to reverse the effects of an overdose of opioids to depress respiration.

Correcting some common misconceptions

Due to the fact that buprenorphine and methadone are opioids, some clinicians have avoided their use and have likened it to merely substituting one opioid for another. So pervasive has been this belief that buprenorphine and methadone have been withheld from many, leading to many attempts by individuals with OUD to repeat re-admissions to inpatient units. Indeed, an abstinence-only philosophy deprives the individual with OUD of a safe, and properly programmed method to manage his or her condition using effective medicinal supplementation.

Whilst individuals without OUD can derive euphoric effects from buprenorphine and methadone, this is seldom the case for those with OUD. This is because chronic OUD leads to desensitization (i.e., less ability to become excited) of opioid receptors, and many individuals with OUD receiving such treatments report feeling no effect and simply a relief from withdrawal symptoms. Maintenance of buprenorphine and methadone is useful in the long-term treatment of OUD because the affected individual can continue with the usual activities of daily life, such as going to school or maintaining employment. Few individuals ever present for treatment because their primary drug of abuse is buprenorphine or methadone.

The slow tapering-off of buprenorphine or methadone, which can take months or years, is the mainstay of treatment. The purpose of medicinal support is not just to provide drugs, but to allow the time rescued by this strategy help the individual to develop other psychosocial supports.

Despite the crisis in OUD, it would be incorrect to propose that most of the prescribed medications, like buprenorphine and methadone, are diverted. In fact, the diversion rate seems to about fifteen percent. Buprenorphine combined with naloxone formulations has been used to decrease diversion, since any attempt to administer the medication intravenously simply results in prominent withdrawal symptoms. This is because if buprenorphine/naloxone is taken in the usual way (i.e., orally), the naloxone moiety is inactive. In contrast, when injected, the naloxone component is active and opposes all agonist opioid actions.

There is a dangerously false belief that individuals administered naloxone for an overdose of opioids are safe immediately, as they become ambulant. Indeed, there are many accounts of overdosed users picked up by an ambulance, administered naloxone, and subsequently becoming ambulant, then jumping out of the ambulance, only to be found dead later on. The reason for this is that naloxone has a short half-life (i.e., stays in the blood only a short time), and it is possible to take enough longer-acting opioids that re-excite the opioid receptors once the naloxone wears off. Truly, this is a tragic result, as being placed in appropriate after-care and monitoring would have prevented calamity.

Even some clinicians confuse detoxification with treatment. Put simply, detoxification is not treatment and, in many cases, is entirely unnecessary, and simple increases the risk of fatality from OUD. This author once read, with absolute horror, a book by a doctor advocating no medicine relief for detoxification as a punishment to deter OUD, i.e., enforce "cold-turkey" (the title of this book has been deliberately withheld). In the Professor's view, this is not only malpractice but torture, which should be punishable as a crime. OUD is a chronic relapsing condition, and appropriate treatment requires medium to long-term supportive medication as well as psychosocial support and proper rehabilitation measures.

Many overdose deaths occur because opioids are combined with other sedative medicines, particularly benzodiazepines and alcohol, which increase their respiratory depressant effects.

Buprenorphine and methadone have significant interactions with other drugs, especially those used to treat HCV and HIV, and must be used with care in individuals with those concomitant conditions. Additionally, those who get HCV whilst on methadone treatment seem to have poorer outcomes, with a greater propensity towards injection drug use. Weaning individuals off methadone too rapidly will increase the risk of illicit opioid injection use, and subsequently, HIV.

Buprenorphine and methadone are essential medicines. Indeed, in 2005, both medicines were included on the list of essential medicines that are "intended to be available within the context of functioning health care systems at all times in adequate amounts, in the appropriate dosage forms, with assured quality, and at a price the individual and the community can afford."

How efficacious is MAT?

Numerous studies have demonstrated the efficacy of methadone in the treatment of OUD. Convincingly, a pivotal meta-analytic review (i.e., many studies combined to determine the overall effect) showed that methadone was more efficacious than placebos even long-term (greater than 6 months) among those receiving psychosocial treatment, and still so when regular counseling services were not provided or available. Methadone use as part of a MAT program resulted in decreased crime and fewer positive opioid-positive drug tests.

Buprenorphine has also been clearly shown to be efficacious as a component of MAT for OUD. OUD individuals who received 16 mg of buprenorphine each day compared with placebo. Whilst the treatment failure rate for buprenorphine was high at 25%, that for the placebo group was 100%. OUD individuals who received buprenorphine, compared with a placebo, were 1.82 times more likely to stay in treatment and had 14.2% fewer urine-positive drug tests. Increasing the maintenance dose of buprenorphine (i.e., greater than 16 mg) is associated with even better outcomes in OUD treatment.

Naltrexone as a daily oral tablet is not the best treatment plan because compliance with the medication tends to be poor. In extended form, extended-release (XR) naltrexone, compared to a placebo, was shown to be associated with 90% vs. 35% abstinent weeks and greater retention (58% vs. 42%, respectively). Naltrexone has the therapeutic disadvantage of requiring detoxification. Nevertheless, in highly motivated individuals with OUD who have been detoxified, the efficacy of XR-naltrexone appears similar to buprenorphine/naloxone combinations.

What MAT regimen works best in pregnant women?

MAT in pregnancy with either methadone or buprenorphine is critical. There is no role or medical rationale for attempting to detoxify a pregnant woman because the medical risks to the mother and fetus are extremely high, and can lead to placental abruption, decreased blood flow to the fetus, premature labor, and death to either and mother and fetus. This does mean that the fetus, when born, will be at risk of Neonatal Abstinence Syndrome (NAS), due to fluctuating and reduced levels of opioids. Such infants need to be supported with methadone, which will be tapered off slowly. Children born with NAS usually have low birth weight, may be premature, and may suffer convulsions. It is important to remember that mothers whose children have developed NAS may have had poor care during pregnancy, and other medical conditions in the mother (e.g., HIV) and child may be masked.

Methadone has been the mainstay of treatment for mothers with OUD since the 1970s. However, the results appear to be more satisfactory with the use of buprenorphine. Using either buprenorphine or methadone will stabilize opioid levels during pregnancy, reduce high-risk behaviors in mothers, and increase the chances of a healthier child being born. It does not make sense to reduce the level of buprenorphine or methadone in pregnancy to avoid NAS since the risk of aberrant and drug-seeking behavior in the mother would most likely result in more challenging or dangerous consequences.

Epilogue

Now, with this background information on OUD and its treatment, you are armed with all the background information needed to understand the subsequent tale. Nevertheless, if you wish for further and more detailed information, there are some really helpful chapters in: *Addiction Medicine*, By Prof.

Dr. Bankole A. Johnson, which was published by Elsevier in 2019.

* * *

Signature Reflection: The Wild Child

Jeremy's story shows how a dragon can grow more than one head: stimulants, gambling, depression, a body under strain. Harrow's compassion does not soften the facts - it sharpens them. The body rings the alarm. The task is to listen before the consequences become irreversible.

If you remember one thing: the body tells the truth before the mind is ready.

- The dragon's disguise: thrill and speed that feel like relief - until they become compulsion.
- The turning point: comprehensive treatment - addressing comorbidity, mood, and behavior, not only the substance.
- A practice to try: identify your early warning sign (sleep, irritability, spending, isolation) and share it with one trusted person.

Clinical lens: neuromodulation tools (like TMS) can be part of care for mood disorders, while addiction recovery often requires layered treatment: psychotherapy, medical monitoring, and relapse-prevention strategy.

We Do Not Need A Superhero!

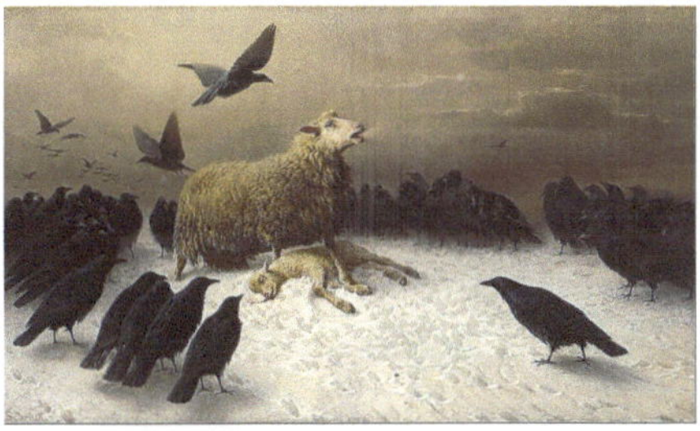

The image above is: "Anguish" - August Friedrich Albrecht Schenk.

In "Anguish", by the German painter August Friedrich Albrecht Schenk (1828-1901), an ewe is depicted crying out in grief over her dead infant surrounded by black crows, the harbinger of death. In our story, Precious is torn apart by the untimely death of her daughter, and her despair is inconsolable. There is only grieving - no healing process going on - and the future, like in the dark skies of the picture, promise no bright future.

This public domain work is in the National Gallery of Victoria, Melbourne.

Superheroes are uniquely American characters. Indeed, we gave birth to them, and they hardly exist in any other culture. Even when they do, it is not to the same extent, and not with so many incredible powers. Superheroes save civilization, avenge the afflicted, fight for justice, and above all, are a comfort to every community that has them.

Psychiatrists and addiction specialists are seldom seen as superheroes in the medical field. That realm of medicine is reserved almost exclusively for surgeons performing heroic tasks (although in John's mind, it is the patients who are superheroes, as they take all the real risks to life and limb). Yet, real superheroes in medicine may be those who devise methods that affect civilizations rather than individual people. If you were to ask John who his superhero is, he would unquestionably answer Dr. Jonas Salk, who invented the polio vaccine. Polio is a crippling disease, and in 1952 at the peak of the epidemic, there were about 58,000 cases, and about 3,000 people died, mostly children. Those who did not die were left with crippling neurological diseases. All Americans remember that Franklin D. Roosevelt got polio at the age of 39 years and was left paralyzed. He later transformed his estate in Warm Springs, Georgia, into a recovery retreat to raise funds to treat patients with polio.

John later drafted these reflections during the first months of the COVID-19 pandemic, when fear moved faster than certainty and the world waited for science to catch up. That moment did not create the truths in this chapter—it simply sharpened them. It reminded him that public health crises do not only test systems; they test the human need to believe, to belong, and to be saved.

John knew the ravages of polio well. His childhood best friend, Ishan, had had polio as a child and was left with half of his body paralyzed. Ishan had few friends. Young boys can be cruel! Other children would not play with him, and he was often to be found sitting gloomily in a corner by himself. Any notion of a girlfriend was out of the question. John enjoyed playing with Ishan, but to his own shame, he sometimes felt it was a burden. John's time with Ishan could not be shared with any other children. Ishan, though, was a courageous man. Despite his occasional gloominess, he maintained a keen sense of looking to the future. He was hopeful that one day there would be a cure for his paralysis, and that his life would resume its intended course...but to date, that has not happened.

John had lost contact with Ishan during his college years and hoped someday to meet with him again. But he was hesitant about where to start, what he might say, and how would he explain the long absence? Failing to resolve this complex but simple emotional dilemma (which could be solved by just picking up the phone and calling) had left John paralyzed with anxiety every time he thought about it. Ergo, nothing got done! Action paralysis.

It was a Friday afternoon at 4 pm many years ago when the fateful call came in through John's assistant. There was someone there to see him who looked "all professional," she said. John knew that anyone hanging around a university at 4 pm on a Friday, who was not actively engaged in research or clinical care, was, by definition, a troublemaker. No administrators in universities plan meetings for late on a Friday afternoon unless they have in mind to fire you. John was hesitant to accept the invitation, but what choice did he have? He was holed up in his office, and his guest knew it.

The man who walked in was the epitome of sartorial elegance, and he was well prepared.

"Mr. John, I am Commodore Herrera, and I am here in my official capacity to ask for you to serve on an important committee to examine how we deliver health care to people addicted to opioids. This is a health emergency. Indeed, the governor should simply declare a state of emergency and put all our efforts together to solve it."

"Just like that?" John quipped.

The man continued, "A health emergency, a rapid response, a long report, and a published solution no one would read or apply. And when all this does not work, the doctors who came up with the "clever" plan are blamed for being too ambitious, and the governor who came up with the idea moves on to his campaign for president as the "strong" man who solved this critical problem. How very nice!".

John was not prone to sarcasm, but he was very afraid. He did not think of himself as a superhero and the burden of the one thousand or so souls he was already looking after weighed heavily on his mind and heart. And now, to add to that, there was a larger undefined problem which would, in all likelihood, result in strategies that required even more time application. It seemed daunting.

So much for work-life balance, John thought.

He regained his posture and formality before speaking. "So, when is this all to start, and how can I help?"

“Yesterday. It’s an emergency,” Horacio replied shortly, with a grin that could only be conjured up by a true expert in the art of human persuasion.

John was glad that his guest was an angel working for the common good.

Had he been recruited by the devil, we would surely all be doomed, and burning up in hell, John mused. “Sign me up,” he said.

John always wished to do good no matter how slim the chances of success and was not worried about being a Captain James Tiberius Kirk on the bridge of The Starship, Enterprise, who always seemed to triumph regardless of the odds. Now he was a superhero! But, John was frightened of becoming *Don Quixote,* whose supposed noble and chivalrous deeds were vanquished by common reality, uncommon sense, and politics.

What transpired over the course of the next 2 years, as John listened to the stories of mothers, fathers, siblings, friends, and yes, children, on his journeys through the State, was beyond politics and left a permanent scar on his heart which he carried as a reminder to the present day.

“Doctor, my name is Precious,” the woman began. Reaching to show him something, she continued. “Here is a picture of my baby girl who we lost just 3 months and 3 days ago.”

John’s mind drifted. He knew that the number 33 was a special number in numerological circles, a rare master number whose set included 11 and 22. The number 33 as an individual usually portended good luck, and represented a personality who usually put the wellness of others above their own affairs, but was him or herself a victim of a fate that could not be changed. John was not a numerologist, he was a scientist, but he had read far and wide and did not believe in coincidences. Something in Precious's story of Angelina would, he believed, come together for him in his understanding of the world.

Precious recounted her story as she rubbed the crucifix around her neck.

"Angelina was my middle child, and she is survived by 2 brothers, each just about 2 years on each side. She was very pretty but fragile in a way that worried us even when she was a child. She could not see the evil in people and was always ready to forgive any transgression. My daughter did well in school and graduated from the University in this state *cum laude* in law. She had everything going for her. She had escaped our humble upbringing, and only the stars were her ceiling. Before she returned home to her native state, Angelina had apprenticed at a prominent law firm in New York. It was there that she had met Franco. Franco was a poor scholar and had only been admitted into the law offices because his father, a prominent real estate broker, had asked a "favor" of his friend who was a partner there.

"Their relationship was odd because they were an odd mixed-race couple, remarkably insensitive to the insensitivity of others. Angelina was always impeccably dressed whilst Franco could not be scruffier. This was not old money dressing down; it was, simply, personal neglect. How on earth could my daughter have fallen for him? Franco had followed her back home like a lap dog, and whilst she had obtained a job in a top law firm, he had mostly developed himself as a professional househusband. But this too was not his calling, and he hardly did any housework, nor did he tend well to any of their affairs. Angelina had a big heart and even forgave his constant philandering. This, however, must have eaten into her core of self-belief and expectation. She felt ruined by Franco but would never leave him.

"On one wintery day, she had fallen off her bicycle and broke her right arm. The fix was easy with a cast, but the hospital's doctor had prescribed 50 oxycodone 10 mg tablets for her to take home and use as she wished, for a period of up to 10 days. At first, Angelina refused to take any medication, but after a sleepless night, worsened by sleeping on their old sofa bed, she took 2 tablets just to get to sleep."

Precious seemed to be pushing down emotions as she paused momentarily.

"I can still remember her call to me the day after her first dose of the tablets. It was as if her world had opened up, and she had become a master of jokes. This was unlike her, and in that flurry of over-excitement as she took more tablets in the coming days. She had opened her heart once more to Franco, and unbeknownst to her, had fallen pregnant. She went through her prescribed medication quickly and returned to her family practitioner for more oxycodone. This time she got a month's supply, and later found out she could get even more by altering her written prescription. Angelina knew this was fraud, and she could be disbarred for it, but who would find out? No one really checked these prescription records properly, and if any problem was found, she would simply deny it. As the pregnancy had advanced, Angelina had begun to miss more and more days at work, and soon the only support she had was unreliable Franco, who had now found himself a young girlfriend - he was done with his brown adventure! The stage was now set for calamity."

John adjusted his position under the tree and motioned for his driver to bring them both some water. It was not a particularly hot day, but it was humid and overcast. A thunderstorm was brewing, and for John, that meant the possibility of a migraine headache. But this was no time or place for him to start popping pills.

"Please continue," John said to Precious.

Tears were now beginning to stream down her face, and her lips looked dry, even after her drink of water. The beauty in her face had been replaced by the dagger of pain, which was now twisting inside of her. John handed over his pocket-handkerchief, leaned forward on the bench, and waited for her to steady herself. With quiet dignity, seemingly born out of the struggle many older black people had faced in America, she continued speaking.

"I did not know much about all this until it was too late. To get more of the medicine into her system, Angelina had started dissolving the oxycodone and injecting it into herself. First in the arm, then the leg, and when she could not find anywhere else that was concealed, between her toes. Eventually, she had sought help as she was worried about the health of the baby. Her family practitioner would not prescribe any medication that could have helped. Although the doctor had read that it was critical to provide a pregnant mother with OUD with medication-assisted treatment (MAT), either buprenorphine or methadone, he had told her to try and simply stop by taking fewer oxycodone tablets. This misguided idea of his was born from something he had read that this would reduce the likelihood of the fetus being addicted. He had not taken into consideration that the health of the mother was intertwined with that of the fetus. Her family practitioner had provided no guidance as to how the oxycodone should be tapered, nor any instructions as to how to get further help. The doctor had, instead, referred her to a local pastor for spiritual guidance, which she attended twice a week.

"The pastor wound up worsening the situation by telling her that MAT was simply substituting one problem for another and that by listening to relaxation tapes and attending the groups, she would find the strength to stop. Angelina could not stay on track with the oxycodone reductions as even small doses declines gave her painful cramps, which she thought would abort the fetus. Additionally, my daughter had not been careful. Franco had started sharing the "fix" and her "works" with her, and she contacted both hepatitis and HIV from him through his new consort. Angelina went into labor after just 25 weeks of pregnancy, but something was badly wrong. Her contractions had started at home, and she thought she would have enough time to get to the hospital. She called 911. A trickle of blood from her vagina had become cups, and after that, it was just a mess by the time she got to the hospital. The doctors at the hospital diagnosed that she had suffered a placental abruption. A caesarian section saved the baby's life, but they had to give her lots of blood to replace what she had lost. Sadly, this led to a dangerously irregular heartbeat (they called it atrial fibrillation), which they could not correct. As if that wasn't enough, she developed another condition called DIC (Disseminated

Intravascular Coagulation, which caused blood clots to occur all over her body. Her organs failed, one at a time, and a couple of hours after arriving at the hospital, my baby passed."

Whilst John was pondering how Precious had remembered all those complicated medical terms (perhaps because it was the only memory of Angelina left to hang on to), Precious' heart burst with agony and grief. She was now screaming as she cried. John had known sadness, but not so suddenly and unexpectedly. John began to sob, and the flood of all the tears he had not shed on the passing of his own mother hit him like a hurricane. John overcame his usual reserve as a physician and hugged Precious. She was not his patient. Precious was another human being in pain, and for John, it was not just the right thing to do, it was the only thing to do.

It seemed like an eternity before Precious and John gathered themselves up again to speak with one another. John recalled that Precious had been rubbing her crucifix and asked about it.

"Are you religious?"

"Yes," she replied.

John, unusually for a scientist physician, was religious and pulled out his mobile phone. His voice stirred.

"I have something I want you to listen to, Precious. Will you bow your head with me? My mother always told me to count my blessings. Now, listen to this as we thank the Lord."

John played Precious one of his most intimate tunes. Indeed, he would request this for his own funeral. It was Mozart's *Laudate Dominum,* sung beautifully and with complete poignance by Tiri Tikanawa.

After a moment dwelling in thought and the song, something occurred to the doctor.

"What happened to the child and Franco?" asked John.

Precious seemed surprised by the question and mumbled her reply.

"I only have an old address for him. And as for Angelina's child, he is that beautiful boy playing over there in the field. His name is Oliver. The doctors at the hospital have been keeping updated and had read some of the work of your team. That's why I wanted to thank you in person. Those doctors did not let Oliver suffer and had given him methadone to ease the pain of not having so much oxycodone on board. Oliver had difficulty in putting on weight - his birth weight was so low - and they brought in a special therapist to help him get comfortable with his feeding bottle. Because his mother had passed, the psychologist had helped Oliver to bond with me, just as if he was my very own."

As John rose to depart, he remembered a song that always inspired him when he felt down.

"Precious, play this whenever you feel down. It's called *You Say* by Lauren Daigle. Believe!" he concluded. John gave Precious a hug and left. They would never meet again, but he would always remember!

Relief for Precious

John had thanked Precious, but before they parted, he arranged for Precious to meet with a psychologist who was a specialist in treating grief reactions. Whilst no one really gets over the death of a child, John was worried that Precious could develop a depressive illness. That psychological team also provided supportive education for the families of those who had an addiction, helping them understand the nature of the disease and why their loved ones just couldn't push the stop button. It was a support group that would enable Precious to understand why the grip of the opioids had paralyzed such a talented, accomplished, and intelligent young woman from seeking help early enough to save herself and her unborn child. In Angelina's case, she died not only of OUD, but of shame. Now think about that; shame as a medical disorder! Finally, the group would enable Precious to grow out of her pain and isolation and be in the best position to mentor Oliver as he grew up, providing her with skills that could protect him from pressures that could lead a path towards addiction.

Precious' story was teaching material suitable for any top-level medical school, but the teaching curriculums for emerging doctors are hard to change and seem to have a penchant for rare and exotic diseases. You would think that addictive disorder, a leading cause of death, would take up months on medical school curriculums, examining every aspect of the disease. Instead, most medical school curriculums in the USA give it just a few weeks. John had lost this battle to change the curriculum, arguing vigorously against recalcitrant deans, but at the end of the day, they were bureaucrats invested in the *status quo*. Their motto seemed to be: 'Do all you can to get to sit on the big can, and when sitting on the can, do as little as possible but look very busy to make sure you do not fall off the can.' Go figure!

The Search for Franco

A few weeks later, John was preparing his suit to go the dry cleaners when he found the crumpled note Precious had given him with Franco's details. How could he have forgotten about that? John realized that he too was processing Precious's grief, and had been angry; indeed blaming Franco for Angelina's death. John felt ashamed at himself and got into his car to try and find Franco.

The old address for Franco was now boarded up, and to be frank, was in such a dangerous part of town that death by opioids would be only one of very many possible ways to meet one's maker in such a place. John got away as fast as he could. He knew some local counselors and shelters in the area that might have taken Franco in.

Sure enough, a few days later, Franco was located, holed up like a rat in a small cardboard shed, abandoned by his own family.

Saving Franco

John enrolled Franco in a MAT program and was started on buprenorphine. A homeless shelter was provided to him, and he became a client of the community outreach counseling group. Franco was no longer using illicit drugs and was on active medication for his HIV. The dose of his buprenorphine had been adjusted to make the anti-retroviral medication for his HIV work effectively. The University, used to personalized care, had made that correction easily.

John came face to face with Franco some 3 months later. Franco had cleaned up and now had a job as a legal assistant. He had been denied access to Oliver until he was 16 years of age, as the social workers and courts had thought it would be too destabilizing. John knew better than to ask Franco 'why'. The man had been on his own journey of despair and was trapped like Angelina in a world he did not want to be. He could not get off this runaway train to anywhere either.

About six months after entering the outpatient OUD program, Franco was finally discharged. He was still taking buprenorphine at a reduced dose, but he seldom had any cravings. His HIV was under control, with no viral activity detected. Perhaps, he was one of the lucky ones! But only time would really tell.

Religion and Science; A Reflection

John had often reflected on the juxtaposition between religion and science. Religion does not stand in the way of science. Faith-based approaches, for those who wish it, might offer solace, comfort, and forbearance. Also, it may enable time for emotional healing.

John, however, saw the treatment of individuals with a chronic brain disorder like OUD to benefit best from a science-based approach. Indeed, the data was clear and unequivocal. Not offering MAT to an individual with an OUD did not make much sense and was simply betting against the patient. In the case of a pregnant mother, for John, not offering MAT in a standardized format was worse than malpractice; it was reckless neglect.

There is a place for faith to support individuals with substance use disorder, but it is not a replacement for evidence-based treatment.

John was troubled by individuals advocating to be treatment providers, with little experience except, perhaps, having been an addict themselves, or simply to extoll their own personal values. Clearly, for John, it was appropriate for the pastor to have offered faith-based support. But when the pastor began advocating against MAT, he had truly crossed the line. John, at first, mused over whether the same pastor would have advocated against treatment for someone with epilepsy? Then, it crossed his mind. Medieval treatments for epilepsy did include the casting out of demons, but this practice, mercifully, is not the mainstay of present treatments. So, why is this the case with addictive diseases? John was left with the numbing conclusion that for practically all disorders that afflicted the brain, which manifested in observable behavioral change, all sorts of religious leaders: shamans, priests, and various religious sects had had their say about what all of it meant in the spiritual world. Truth be told, the curse of addiction remains not in the nature of the brain disease, but in the many obstacles to obtaining proper evidence-based treatment. Regulations were few, and repercussions for the practitioner of bad medicine were rare. What other fields of medicine reward the failure of the practitioner so handsomely by the patient returning to spend even more money to seek treatment?

Thanking Horacio

It was precisely 4.01 pm on a Friday when John was ushered into Horacio's office. Horacio had the same grin on him as he did when they met a couple of years earlier. John thought the grin must have been painted on him as part of his superhero costume, but there was no cape.

"Congratulations on the hard work, John. I have a commendation to you signed by the governor," Horacio said.

He could not resist continuing, "And he's running for President next fall. Who would have guessed?"

John accepted his letter of commendation gracefully and

headed to the door. On his way, he turned around to add, "Thank you for getting me out of my mind paralysis! I really thought I had seen it all, but this experience has taught me that life is new, we only never stop for long enough to notice it!"

As John fired up his inspirational 12-cylinder British car and roared down the road, there was only one song to play - Tina Turner's *We Don't Need Another Hero*. Tina's own story of despair, being trapped, and finally, glorious redemption is a lesson for us all to cherish.

Ten Days

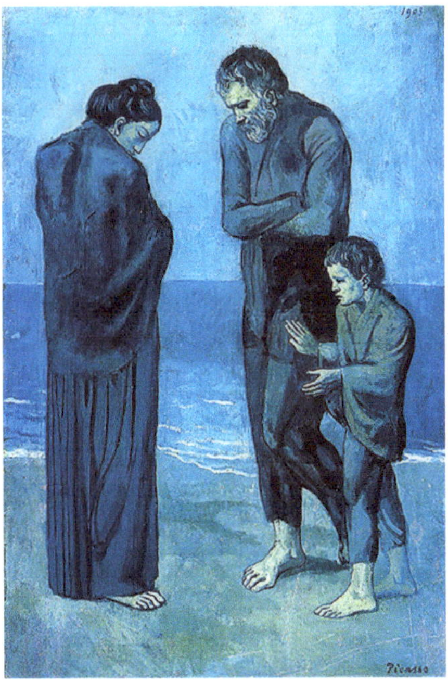

The image above is: 1903 painting by Pablo Picasso.

In this 1903 picture painted by Pablo Picasso, there are three characters in desolation and despair. The use of the color blue in this painting is to depict sadness, gloom, and foreboding. The absence of an actual scene of tragedy ensures that the viewer remains transfixed and does not avert the eye or recoil in revulsion.

In this story, there are three characters, one man, a boy, and a girl. Allegorical to the characters in the story, they too are stranded in despair associated with opioid use, and there is no boat in sight to take them to safety. As in this story, the characters do not seem to be related but are somehow acquainted, perhaps chained together by their fate. All in all, this is a haunting picture, which is reminiscent of John's tale, and his own present history of loss - again with three characters - his mother, father, and ex-fiancé.

John's haunting began at precisely 10 pm on the evening of October 4, 1982. He had just returned from burying his father, who died just six short weeks after his mother, both of terminal cancer. John did not believe in coincidences, so the seed of doubt that resided in his mind was inescapable. John was not himself, and indeed, he wasn't anyone else he knew either. On that same wet night in Glasgow, his fiancé had informed him she was leaving to be with a much wealthier friend, who could promise her a life of great ease and luxury. As he bid her goodbye, his phone rang.

John had been called in to the hospital as there was a shortage of doctors; many had refused to come in on account of having the flu. Never one to shirk a challenge, John had climbed into his car, the wipers seemingly wiping his tears rather than the windscreen, and drove the short 5-mile trip to the hospital. He was on automatic pilot, and the symbolism of the day had escaped his memory. It was not like him.

One of the mysteries of being a young doctor was that the lesson of working out who the patient was had not been learned. As John walked into the emergency room that evening, he was directed to see a young girl who had been brought in by a middle-aged, dark-haired man, who was wearing a pair of khaki shorts. On any given day, John would have noticed the incongruity of this presentation except that he was distracted by the young girl writhing on the bed, eyes rolling towards the back of her head, tongue protruding, and her voice letting out a gentle cry as her neck contorted uncontrollably. Her face was remarkable for what looked like grimacing of the jaw, and this presentation, reminiscent of a young girl in a horror movie seemingly possessed by a demonic presence, was alarming indeed.

John turned to the nurse by his side, who was still recoiling in shock at what she was witnessing and shouted, "10 mg of intravenous benztropine stat!" The nurse, true to her training, snapped out of her blank gaze and infused the medicine into a catheter in the young girl's veins. "Wait for it, 1 min countdown," screamed John as a crowd of other doctors had raced in. "Don't touch her, just wait," he followed as he set the chronometer on his mechanical wristwatch. Almost on cue, the young girl stopped her movements, sat up calmly, and hugged her father. The other doctors gave John a knowing nod. It's not often that the psychiatry intern is the hero in an emergency room. That role was always seemingly reserved for the surgeons, who are always seen running around the emergency room, stemming the bleeding of limbs, or physicians bring back a patient to life by applying the electric shock pads of life. Many other doctors would have confused the girl's condition for an epileptic seizure. But not John, even in his emotionally flooded mind.

Relieved, John took a chair next to the bed and turned to the girl's father to get a history. Of course, John had worked out the correct diagnosis - an oculogyric crisis - but no one had seen a reaction so severe in any patient, let alone a teenager. Even more shockingly, she was too young to be on strong medicines known as antipsychotics that could have caused this. This stems from the fact that antipsychotics are prescribed to people with severe mental illness. The teenager, Julie, had been traveling with her older brother, Scott, and their father from the highlands. The twisty and bumpy roads had not been kind to Julie, and she had been overcome by motion sickness. Her father, Mr. Gregory, had come prepared for the trip, or so he thought, and had given her two 25 mg tablets of a medicine called metoclopramide, which had produced her symptoms, and which were subsequently cured by the simple antidote. In his panic to give Julie the medicine, her father had not noticed that half of the tablets in the bottle were missing. Strangely also, for some reason, John had forgotten to ask how many tablets were left in the bottle. John's simple oversight would come back to haunt him! Somehow, no one had noticed that Julie's brother, Scott, had an unsteady gait as he walked to hug both his sister and father.

John stayed in the hospital overnight, and as he made his way to take his shower at 7 am, his pager went off. "Horror of horrors" John had muttered under his breath. He had not had much sleep and was looking forward to getting home, if only to digest all that had happened in his own life over the last month. Seeing a patient at 7 am was just trouble. There was no chance of getting off at 8 am as scheduled, not with all the notes and entries that had to be made, and worse, if it got complicated, he could be there till noon. Gamely, John responded to his pager and shuffled slowly back into the emergency room. He did not feel like a hero now, just another over-worked young doctor. And guess who his next patient was: same old Mr. Gregory. However, this time, it was Scott who seemed to be needing attention. John mused to himself, it was day 2, and another member of Mr. Gregory's family was his patient. What lay in store for day 3, Mrs. Gregory, Mr. Gregory, the whole family? Indeed, who was the patient in greatest need? All he was being presented with were emergent symptoms in each family member.

Scott had a pasty look about him, and his short brown hair was matted against his forehead with sweat. He was holding his stomach as if in pain, and he was sobbing and in tears. Scott recounted that his bowels were loose but what truly gave it all away were his widely dilated pupils. How was this a consult for the psychiatric intern and not the acute medical team? It was simply protocol. Since John had seen one family member, and had supposedly built a rapport with the rest of them, it made sense for him to be asked to see another family member who had been involved in the same incident. However, were these the same incidents or were they different? John took a careful history, and this time, he did remember to ask about how many tablets of metoclopramide were left in the bottle. Scott turned red with embarrassment as everyone's gaze turned to him. He unfolded his arms to reveal a scab covering a recent puncture wound. Scott, at the young age of 19 years, was a heroin addict, and his symptoms were those of opioid withdrawal. What a shock! Well, at least the treatment for this condition was clear as day. As Scott was not throwing up, John ordered 40 mg of methadone for him to drink, which seemed to calm down his withdrawal symptoms. But this was not treatment - just a quick fix in the emergency! John admitted Scott to the hospital to stay until he could be seen later on by an addiction specialist to receive medication-assisted treatment for his heroin addiction. John was furious with himself. How had he not asked about how many tablets of metoclopramide had been left in the bottle? Perhaps he would have figured out that Scott had been using the medicine to stop his nausea when he injected himself with heroin? Well, no great harm had been done, and at least, he had got it right in the end. So John thought.

Day 3, and John was relaxing at home when his phone rang. It was Doctor Stromberg, his colleague, on the phone. He had heard of John's interactions with the Gregory family and was calling to follow up. "John, we had an interesting evening with Scott. He took his methadone alright, and we referred him to an outpatient center for further treatment. He has refused to go, saying that giving him methadone is just a crutch and he would rather just wing it on his own. Please can you come and talk him out of it," said Dr Stromberg. John groaned. Somehow, he wasn't quite getting all to fit with this case, and it gave him an uncomfortable feeling. "Of course," replied John, who quickly darted to his car to see Scott. By the time he got to the hospital, Scott had discharged himself against medical advice and was nowhere to be found. A call to his father also proved fruitless. Indeed, Mr Gregory's phone, which no one had had the good sense to test, was no phone at all but a pager. How very strange! Well, not much could be done about it except to ask the local social services to try and follow up. As Scott was of legal age and was classified as having an addiction, he could not be detained involuntarily under the Mental Health Act. In any case, that would have been counterproductive, as he would only have been released upon further assessment, and the treatment given for of addiction is that of a chronic disease.

Day 4, and John had returned to his usual duties in the emergency room. It was a quiet night, except for a few people turning up to mend their cuts and sprains from some scrap they had gotten themselves into earlier. Then, that foghorn no one loves to hear came from the speakers in the ER and was closely followed by an announcement "incoming vehicular accident, 3 victims, 2 men and one girl. Everyone to their stations". John grabbed his stethoscope, tourniquet, and ophthalmoscope, and rushed to incident room # 1. On entering, John almost fell over with shock. It was Mr Gregory. Like a man turning over the page in a horror story, John took a peek at room # 2 and then room # 3. "Oh no!" he exhaled sharply. It was the Gregory family, and from what he could see, all seemingly in the same clothes as when he had first met them! There wasn't much that could be done for Mr Gregory or Julie - they'd lost too much blood! John hurriedly worked with the other doctors to do all they could for Scott. It was touch and go for an hour, and John had never seen anyone lose so much blood within such a short space of time.

Days like this test everything you believe in, not just your religion.

Day 5, John got up early to visit Scott at the hospital. He was hoping that his would be a familiar face for him to see once he woke up from his sedation. It was the least he could do, he thought. But Scott was not improving. Apparently, he had discharged himself from the hospital just to "score". And by that act he had done so many times before without incident, he sealed his fate. When he was brought back in, Scott was running a temperature of 104 degrees Fahrenheit and had cooling blankets on. He had injected bacteria into his own body, causing a massive septic reaction. John knew that not much more could be done, and he knelt beside Scott's bed to say a prayer. It was a prayer his mother had taught him to sing "O God, our help in ages past..." from Psalm 90, the first chronological Psalm attributed to Moses. It was a hope for a longer life. Scott fought hard, but on the tenth day from their first meeting (i.e. Day 10), he died.

John attended the postmortem, which was quite revealing. Mr Gregory was not the father of Julie and Scott. In fact, they were his pushers, and Mr Gregory was a dealer. Julie's story of using metoclopramide for car sickness also was not true. She, too, was addicted to opioids and was taking the metoclopramide to quell the subsequent nausea from the incessant abuse of drugs. But because she was not injecting, there were no tell-tale track marks to give away the real diagnosis. The giveaway in the presentation were the shorts Mr. Gregory had been wearing. Why would anyone on a cold and wet day in later autumn in Glasgow be wearing shorts? Actually, Mr. Gregory had been at home when all this happened and had made up the story when Julie was brought to the emergency room.

John and his colleagues learned this lesson the hard way. It was not their fault but the question as to who was the real patient, rather than just the person in front of them with symptoms, was the unanswered question. John learned that for his part, something that would help him some 20 years later, was to always ask about the health of all those who came with the patient and not make any assumptions. John would never forget that day for another good reason. It fell exactly 400 years at the end of the Julian calendar (October 4, 1582), which was followed by 10 uncounted days before the beginning of the Gregorian calendar, which we still use today. And as for coincidence, that really does not exist for John. Not the date, and not even that the central patient called Mr Gregory. All were clues. If John had been superstitious, he would have thought them a premonition. Everything has its own order, and we are drawn to all things by a set of forces we do not understand.

John reflected deeply from his experience, which put his own grief into perspective. Just because you think you are having the worst of it does not mean that others are not having a more terrible time. John again heard his mother's voice in his head whispering "count your blessings one by one..."

Chapter 10

Some Concluding Remarks To Book 2 of 3

You've reached the end of Book 2 - where the science becomes more intricate, and the hope becomes more specific.

Many of these allegorical stories unfold years before the present, because personalization is not a trend - it is a long, disciplined pursuit of understanding what makes each person unique.

This volume is the most technically dense in the series. But the purpose of the science is simple: to reduce suffering by improving precision.

John appears at times, but he is not the sole teacher here. The cast widens, because real learning often comes through others - mentors, patients, colleagues, and even adversaries.

As you move through the chapters, notice what changes in the characters: not just what they know, but what they value, what they fear, and what they are willing to face.

The final story anchors us in the past and then gently

pivots - setting the stage for a return to the present, where stressors are louder and the stakes feel higher.

Book 3 will take you into that world: awareness under pressure, reactivity under strain, and the possibility of elevation - even in the midst of crisis.

Read on.

Chapter 11

Further Reading and References

Johnson BA, Roache JD, eds. *Drug addiction and its treatment: nexus of neuroscience and behavior*. Philadelphia, PA: Lippincott-Raven Publishers; 1997.

Johnson BA, Ruiz P, Galanter M, eds. *Handbook of clinical alcoholism treatment*. Baltimore: Lippincott Williams & Wilkins; 2003.

Johnson BA, ed. *Addiction medicine: science and practice*. New York: Springer Science+Business Media; 2010.

Johnson BA, Roache JD, Javors MA, DiClemente CC, Cloninger CR, Prihoda TJ, Bordnick PS, Ait-Daoud N, Hensler J. Ondansetron for reduction of drinking among biologically predisposed alcoholic patients: a randomized controlled trial. *JAMA*. 2000;284:963-971.

Johnson BA, Ait-Daoud N, Bowden CL, DiClemente CC, Roache JD, Lawson K, Javors MA, Ma JZ. Oral topiramate for treatment of alcohol dependence: a randomized controlled trial. *Lancet*. 2003;361:1677-1685.

Johnson BA, Rosenthal N, Capece JA, Wiegand F, Mao L, Beyers K, McKay A, Ait-Daoud N, Anton RF, Ciraulo DA, Kranzler HR, Mann K, O'Malley SS, Swift RM, Topiramate for Alcoholism Advisory Board, Topiramate for Alcoholism Study Group. Topiramate for treating alcohol dependence: a randomized controlled trial. *JAMA*. 2007;298:1641-1651.

Anton RF, O'Malley SS, Ciraulo DA, Cisler RA, Couper D, Donovan DM, Gastfriend DR, Hosking JD, Johnson BA, LoCastro JS, Longabaugh R, Mason BJ, Mattson ME, Miller WR, Pettinati HM, Randall CL, Swift R, Weiss RD, Williams LD, Zweben A, COMBINE Study Research Group. Combined pharmacotherapies and behavioral interventions for alcohol dependence - The COMBINE Study: a randomized controlled trial. *JAMA*. 2006;295:2003-2017.

Johnson BA, Ait-Daoud N, Seneviratne C, Roache JD, Javors MA, Wang X-Q, Liu L, Penberthy JK, DiClemente CC, Li MD. Pharmacogenetic approach at the serotonin transporter gene as a method of reducing the severity of alcohol drinking. *Am J Psychiatry*. 2011;168:265-275.

Johnson, BA. Addiction Medicine. Published by Elsevier, 2019

BOOK 3: Awareness, Reactivity, and Elevate

Chapter 12
Introduction To Book 3 Of 3

In Book 3, the narrative pauses in the COVID era—a season when the world held its breath. From that pressure-cooker, John looks backward again, letting the earlier years speak with new clarity, and carrying their lessons forward into what comes next.

A viral pandemic spreads, but another crisis gathers underneath: the mental health aftershock - fear, isolation, grief, and the strain of uncertainty.

The social distancing meant to protect bodies can starve the nervous system of connection. Stress-related conditions rise, and old coping strategies become tempting again.

At the same time, tensions around injustice, poverty, and instability intensify. For many, the pressure is not theoretical - it is daily.

Here, John returns in fuller force. He is not only observing the crisis; he is preparing to meet it, on the front lines of the mind.

He also knows how much remains unknown: how a novel virus may affect the brain, how trauma accumulates, and how resilience can be built when resources are scarce.

Against the "life must go on" mantra, the book explores what it takes to keep going without losing yourself - how to respond rather than react.

Some characters are quarantined, trapped in hotel rooms with their thoughts. Others are trapped in patterns they've repeated for years. Either way, the setting becomes a laboratory for change.

For John, this volume is emotionally demanding. It pulls him back into childhood memories, even as it pushes him toward a more expansive understanding of adulthood.

This book deepens the foundations of brain wellness introduced in Book 1, showing how stress, relationships, and meaning can either erode - or elevate - our health.

It also brings forward conversations about sexual behavior and related disorders that often complicate recovery, yet are too often ignored.

New knowledge can be medicine. When you understand what is happening inside you, shame loosens - and choice returns.

John is awake, and the stories are ready. So are you.

Towards the next series!

"...beyond science...beyond borders ***TM****"*

Awareness And Reactivity

The Sword of Damocles

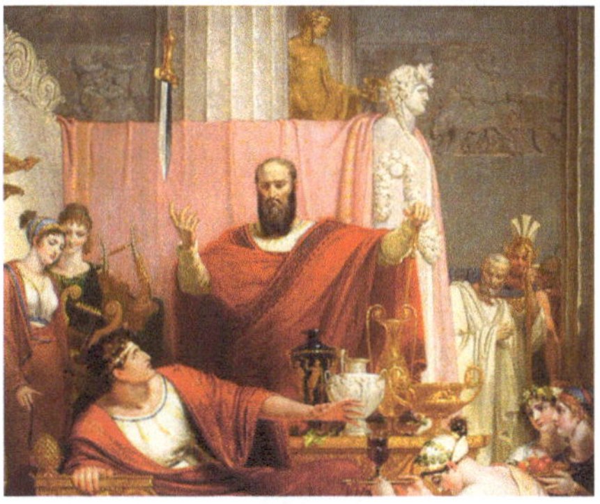

The image above depicts Richard Westall's Sword of Damocles.

In modern times, the sword of Damocles depicts a feeling of foreboding or gloom. In ancient times, however, from the writings of Cicero (106 - 43 BC), the Sword of Damocles is a story that interweaves tyranny with high educational refinement. It is a warning of not prejudging people's intentions by their manifest behavior. The roots of the story hark even further back to the court of Dionysius, a tyrant of the 4th century. Damocles was a flatterer of Dionysius's great wealth and power so much that Dionysius implored Damocles to exchange places with him. Damocles was feasted and heralded with beautiful attendants, lavish food, and glorious incense was burned. Yet, above Damocles's head hung a sword held by only a single horsehair to remind him of the peril of leadership. Damocles begged Dionysius to exchange places back stating that he preferred his impoverished life to one with the constant peril of impending death despite being surrounded by riches. Dionysius is often confused as one person in folklore even though there was an elder and a younger. Consistent with the addiction theme of this book, the elder Dionysius was famed with inviting two drunks who spoke ill of the king. He then plied them with wine, and the one with the "looser" tongue was let go as his folly was solely attributable to alcohol abuse. The other, who was more reserved and careful was put to death as a true traitor as he betrayed the king in full consciousness. The younger Dionysius fared little better than his elder brother and was famous for living a life of debauchery for which he blamed being the son of a tyrant.

Pertinent to our story, John is faced with the peril of a life and death struggle for his soul, understanding, and professional life. Like the tale of the Sword of Damocles, his choices appeared to be limited; yet he finds a way. Allegorical to John's story, and the ancient tale, is not only the inevitability that this question of a pivotal decision must be answered at some time in life, but that tyranny had its "roots" in an earlier generation. Tyranny begets the same. John's understanding of Ian's predicament is based on the link between the past and the present. Cicero's tale is at pains to remark that cruelty also might be discharged by the highly educated. Additionally, Cicero's tale, like our story, is a warning that those with power labor under the constant specter of anxiety and apprehension, and that this stress is the progenitor of a great primordial unhappiness, often stemming from childhood, for which a cure is hard to find. Only by driving through this pain and working through its re-emergence can there be solace.

For a further analysis of the Sword of Damocles, see "What did Cicero mean by the Sword of Damocles

The old image of the sword overhead is useful because it is honest: even a good life can feel unsafe when the blade is always present. In this Signature Edition's language, When Dragons Kill, they often do it through unrelenting stress - quietly teaching the brain to trade long-term health for short-term relief.

When stress becomes chronic, it narrows the mind. It shortens the distance between cue and reaction. It makes relief feel urgent - and that urgency can be the doorway through which substances, compulsions, and self-sabotage enter.

Stress is not only what happens to you; it is what your nervous system predicts is about to happen. It is the body rehearsing danger, again and again, until rehearsal feels like reality.

Harrow's Field Note: Stress as a Hanging Blade

Stress is the trilogy that unites the past, present, and future. It is the reincarnation of the incomplete, which can never be resolved at its root but poses two chimeras for salvation in the present or future. There is always a choice!

Stress is an infection that permeates all that it comes into contact with, sits by the side in mocking hibernation, only to re-emerge at an inopportune time, when even more is going wrong to rankle the soul.

Like dust, stress attracts more of itself, such that seemingly unrelated matters become intertwined into an inarticulate jumble. Once the stress infection truly sets in, just like a microbe, it delivers its toxicity with quick dispatch in an attempt to kill its host.

Using the wrong medicine or therapy to abate stress, or not enough of the right ones, can make the situation worse as more of the stress infection is now liberated from its previous containment, to overwhelm the entire being. At that point, curing the sepsis of stress is hard as it takes on new names to disguise its roots like depression, traumatic disorder, and the like, antidotes are not readily found, and the path to wellness is long, weary, complicated, and you guessed it, laden with even more potential for stress.

Stress can kill, and frequently does!

In the early months of COVID-19 (2020), when the air felt heavy with uncertainty and the news carried a daily tally of loss, John found himself rereading old notebooks from his formative years. He remembered what it had taken to free himself from the tyrannical trilogy of stress—not as a heroic conquest, but as a practiced refusal to let fear write the script of his life.

In those notes, one season stood out: John had been on sabbatical, having sought the mentorship of a stout but roguish looking but preening scientist, called Ian Mackintosh. Ian reminded John, in many ways by character, of all his own father's faults that he had later came to forgive.

Ian was a notable and astute scholar, and word had it that he was next in line for the most vaunted prize in science. John had not processed why he was so interested in this sabbatical, as he was at the height of his career, and really did not need anymore "training". But, at heart, John was a scholar, and surely there was something new he could learn from another of such esteem.

In his laboratory, Ian was disliked by all. He was a bully and tyrant, although he did not seem to know it or simply did not care. Ian's worn and leather-like character was impervious to either observation or change. Or so it seemed. Indeed, he was seldom ever in his laboratory, and when he did show up, made quite a song and dance of it all to announce his presence. Simply, it was tiring. John hated pretense, especially when wrapped in pride and arrogance.

John recalled a particularly distressing meeting with Ian who had returned to the laboratory after a week away giving lectures. It was a cold and icy day, and John had done all he could to be no more than 5 min late (six being his cut-off for carelessness or rudeness). Unfortunately for John, Ian who was typically almost 45 min late had arrived on time and was lying in wait fuming under his breath. Ian was in a foul mood, obviously stressed by something that had happened earlier, and was going to “let John have it”, justified or not. “John”, Ian howled, “I have a story to tell you today about being late that will change the course of your life”. John was all ears; he really wasn’t late at all. Indeed, it had not escaped John’s attention that Ian’s wall clock in his office was an hour and five minutes fast, not having been corrected for wintertime. How truly careless for someone about to give a lecture on timeliness! Ian continued to bellow, “a few years ago, I was traveling to give a lecture at an ivy league school in the Mid-West. I was proud to be giving that lecture, and my teenage son was accompanying me. As we approached the bridge, across which was the university, there was a huge roadblock, and you could see a stream of police cars and fire engines up ahead. If I had sat in that traffic, I would have been very late. So, I unfastened my seat belt, asked my teenage son to take over, leapt out of the car and ran across the bridge”. John was jogged into disbelief and waited to hear Ian say that he arrived on time. But no. Ian continued excitedly - “I got there 20 min late and my lecture had been cancelled. But it felt great that I had made such a bold attempt to get there on time. It’s called commitment. Of course, the lecture had to be rescheduled but my apology when I did give the lecture was met with applause as I recounted my previous attempt to be there. Character building! What do you think of that John? Lesson learned?”.

John understood that he was being baited but was more intrigued by the reasoning that had brought Ian to making, as he saw it, a flawed set of ever more dangerous decisions. Furthermore, John was on sabbatical, and could have left anytime, but such was Ian’s reputation that he didn’t wish to upset him, especially if it could be avoided by guile. John clenched his teeth hard. So much so that part of his cheek got caught between his teeth and it began to bleed. John could smell that unmistakable scent of fresh blood as it inflamed the back of his throat and nostrils.

John hated the smell of blood! It was like death.

During his training as an intensive care specialist about three decades earlier, he had worked on an emergency surgical team. It was the first day of July, the most dangerous day in Christendom for medical care. It was the first day the young surgical residents were unleashed on real patients. John recalled rushing to the operating theater on that fateful day about three decades ago. A middle-aged man had been brought into theater with a knife stuck in his abdomen. He had quarreled with his wife and had gone out to get drunk in the pub. Returning in the early hours of the morning, he had crawled through the kitchen window so as not to awaken his presumably still irate wife. Believing her husband to be an intruder, she had stabbed him in the abdomen. The wound looked sinister and the knife throbbed back and forth in the patient's abdomen. Even the young John knew that an experienced surgeon was needed, and he pleaded with the new surgical resident to call the senior supervising surgeon. The new surgical resident refused, and John, doing his duty escorted the patient to theater and put him under anesthesia. It did not take long for the surgical resident to yank the knife out of the patient's abdomen. Bloodshot from the damaged vessel, splattered on the ceiling, fanned out, then spread downward like a shower of engorged wet dust particles. Even more blood burbled out from the open wound like an overflowing river. Blood was everywhere! John had climbed on to the operating table to apply pressure on the wound with his left hand, and at the same time he had used his right hand to apply a set of metal clamps to shut off the pumping head of blood. John knew that the patient had suffered a puncture to his abdominal aorta and that pulling out the knife suddenly was truly a very bad idea. The pump head of blood stopped only to be followed by a diffuse oozing of more of the red stuff. Twenty liters of blood and fluids were infused over several hours into the patient, but the oozing continued. The patient had developed a terrible condition called disseminated intravascular coagulation, whereby the blood oozing out of the patient's blood vessels would not form a clot, and even when the blood did clot, it broke apart into small friable pieces, which when transmitted to his organs as emboli, caused them to fail. John was desperate to save the patient, and so was the rest of the team, but it was hopeless. The patient expired! That was the last time John worked with a surgical team. The very next day, John informed his superiors that he could not take the recklessness of young surgeons, which would be repeated each year, and he transitioned to his present career as a mental health specialist.

Now, the echo of that strong smell of blood from decades ago, collided with John's present, invoked flashbacks in John, and induced him into an uncomfortable dream-like state. That was the echo that had travelled back to the first part of John's trilogy of stress and was now in the present.

John's dream-like detached state was interrupted by what sounded like a distant foghorn of a voice. "Go on, tell me what you really think John, after all you're just here on sabbatical, just us two chatting like grown-ups". Again, John hesitated. In John's mind's eye, Ian was more likely to have been brought down by a hail of bullets from the policemen on the other side of the bridge than reach his destination. Perish the thought. Just another example of recklessness in the here and now, like that day three decades ago in the surgical theater. It was all John could stand! Yet, he was composed enough to remain compassionate. Even Ian would not have deserved the fate of being plunged into perdition's flame! John could not be more out of his mind with stress! All this that was now transpiring straight out of Hamlet Act 3 Scene 1 (where Hamlet debates whether or not to avenge the death of his murdered father by killing his murderer) in so many of its parts not just the first line that most are apt to repeat or quote. To John, here were the important elements: "*To be or not to be: that is the question: Whether 'tis nobler in the mind to suffer the slings and arrows of outrageous fortune, or to take arms against a sea of troubles, and by opposing end them?...the insolence of office...the patient merit of the unworthy takes, when he himself might his quietus make... thus conscience does make cowards of us all...and lose the name of action*". In that soliloquy, Hamlet's past is brought forwards into the present, which would determine his future. It was, the trilogy of stress!

John was in no doubt. He was now facing the "true death" not in terms of his mortality but as to whether he could remold his past demons, to secure the present, and move into the future. Like in Hamlet's soliloquy, John was aware that he faced the conundrum of the trilogy. John was aware that in this present, he could kill his own self-esteem by letting the past dominate his future. He bit harder into his cheek. John was cognizant enough to realize that his "quietus" (a legal Latin term meaning a definitive termination to an argument) also could symbolize by inaction, a kind of cowardice in and of itself. This was not passing through the trilogy but being caught in it like an insect in a spider's web. John knew that it would be bat-hit crazy to give into his demons and aggrandize Ian with a reply.

John got up from his seat and feigned a swoon. Ian got up to catch him and called in his assistant to bring in some water. In the commotion of that moment, John had avoided an answer to the question. He had ducked the bullet. John would never allow himself to be baited into a no-win scenario.

On his way back after the meeting, John reflected on what had actually happened. It is obvious that Ian's father was an abusive parent and must have punished him for any tardiness. As Ian's esteem had grown as a scientist, and he now was in a position of power, he now used his own notorious lateness to abuse others. Ian's stressful childhood had not only germinated but had borne poisonous fruit that was now dispatched to any unsuspecting passerby. But as this was personal, the poison had to be passed on to a reflection of himself in some manner. Ergo, John!

John understood Ian's unrelenting pain. It was an unquenchable thirst. Indeed, Ian had placed himself in a psychological no-win situation on the bridge that day. None of this would have made immediate sense to a casual observer.

But John was no casual observer. Ian's race across the bridge into untold danger, and possible death, as who could tell whether the armed police on the opposite side of the bridge with pistols drawn were seeking someone of anything of Ian's description fleeing from justice, was, as in Hamlet's soliloquy, "*the undiscovered country*". In Hamlet, the *undiscovered country* was death, which could possibly be more terrifying than life itself, and most certainly worse as there would then be no means of changing the present reality. Ian leaving his teenage son in the car to fend for himself, and face the unknown, was unthinkable to John. John had met Ian's son and knew he could hardly drive. Ian leaving his teenage son in the car was part of the same plot of "helplessness" that he had infected him with both psychologically and in reality. The paralysis of stress! The trilogy had been passed on from Ian to his teenage son!

John reflected on how he had come to forgive his own father. He had come to realize that his father's choices were out of a set of circumstances that had locked him in, and he had made choices as best he could, bouncing between the past and the present, and had continued to make them, sometimes alternatively trying to change the outcome, but with no hope of escaping to a better future.

As a child, John had often been challenged by his own father. John was barely 7 years of age whereupon his father had asked him to play a game of chess with him. John would rather have played soccer with his friends and boasted to his father that he could beat him blindfolded. John's father was incensed and the young John, now blindfolded, was forced to play his father at chess. John's father lost the game, smashed the chess pieces, and hardly spoke with him ever again. John had lost that no win scenario. That was the primordial stress in John's trilogy. Surely, the John of today would never have allowed himself to be placed in that position and had learned that lesson well. He dreamt often that, now in the present, he could go back to that day and "fix it" and tell his father how much he loved him. John would not have thrown the game of chess on purpose but would have found some way to ease by the situation. Sometimes, you can refuse to be either the reed that bends with the wind, or the immovable stone by simply not being there! No need to be ensnared by the spider-web of bad decisions. John knew that had the roles been reversed with his father, he would scream with joy if either of his sons prevailed against him in any game, and celebrate their victory with all his heart, like it was the best day on earth.

John's salvation that day in Ian's room was that he wherewithal to remove himself from being an actor in this scripted Shakespearean play, and to create his own reality. In doing so, he had accepted that like anyone else, he too, could be a victim of the trilogy of stress but had chosen not to be. John was free!

Several months later, at the end of his sabbatical, John decided to write to Ian.

"My Dear Ian,

I start by wishing both you and your family well and shall look forward to the promise of our meeting again.

Several months ago, you had posed to me this conundrum of your time on the bridge and your attempt to get to a lecture on time that you did not wish to miss.

I was unable to answer you at that time, as all I could feel was your pain, and any lesson to be learned was in my own inability to accept you as who you are.

For that, you have my deepest apology.

I was lost in the stress of my own pain and had to claw my way out.

You might wish to read Hamlet Act 3 scene 1 to understand my own dilemma at that time, but that may just feel to you like an intellectual exercise. I promise you that it is not. Instead, it is a moral dilemma of accepting ourselves that we all must face, sometimes, many times in a lifetime.

For me, that pain of getting to know myself come as a trilogy - once as a child, then as a young doctor, and that day in your office.

For you, it would seem that you have failed to answer this question, even now, but I know not when you were first presented with it.

I can share, that like you, I had a difficult time growing up, with huge expectations. It was truly rough, and perhaps, I do what I do now just because of that. Indeed, I did meet those expectations full on, and worked through my pain. The cost of not doing so would have been too high.

On the day my father died, although we had not shared any true emotions for most of my life, I wept like a child so as to bring about my being able to forgive him.

Nevertheless, it took me thirty years from the day he died to forgive myself.

Now, I pray for my father to forgive me, and yours you, so that the cycle of pain will truly end with this generation; for yours and my sake.

The past, the present, and the future need not all be the same. Fused, together in the spell of fate.

I have told my own children the story of that meeting with you many times, not as a nightmare to be recounted, but as a sentinel to always guide them away from the Sword of Damocles that pivots between the present and the future, as the past cannot be altered. Only how we feel about it, or look back at it.

In closing, I wish to assure you that I did learn the lesson well. Not that which you intended, but instead, that which, I hope, has allowed us to both move forward.

We must own our past, bring it into the present, and strive to do all we can to enter the "undiscovered country". Therein, we will hope to find the fountain of true wellness at the end of the rainbow.

Ever,

Professor John Horacio Harrow."

Two weeks later, on just another Thursday afternoon, John was browsing restlessly on his computer as if hunting for a question without an answer. Flashed across was an email he had just received from the College headed "Important announcement". John read it quickly:

"*We are sad to announce the death of Professor Ian Mackintosh. His wife described his last weeks as his best. Ian had mustered the energy to give the annual commencement speech remotely, whereupon he spoke about the power of forgiveness, getting to know his brother again who had moved back to Israel two decades earlier, and how the pain of the soul surpassed any he had felt from his cancer. In that lecture, he had described himself as having started his life as if pursued by a black crow only to be coming to its end being buzzed by hummingbirds. In lieu of flowers, please donate any gifts to the World Health Organization COVID-19 Solidarity*

Response Fund With gratitude for a life well lived, his enduring partner, Emily Mackintosh"

Ian's trilogy was complete. His haunting past had somehow been resolved in the present, even though the future was short. But it was different! The Trilogy was complete.

* * *

Signature Reflection: The Sword of Damocles

Under the hanging sword, Ian learns what many of us postpone: the nervous system relaxes when unfinished relational business is addressed. The story turns foreboding into clarity - grief, forgiveness, and reconciliation as acts of strength rather than sentiment.

If you remember one thing: peace is not passive - it is chosen.

- The dragon's disguise: success that hides chronic dread.
- The turning point: speaking the truth in time - repairing what can be repaired while life is still available.
- A practice to try: one honest message. Name what matters, without theatrics. Then press send.

Clinical lens: unresolved conflict keeps stress physiology activated. Repair and meaning-making can lower the baseline

- improving sleep, mood, and the capacity to tolerate uncertainty.

Field Note (2020): The Curious Story of George and the Coming Post-COVID Era

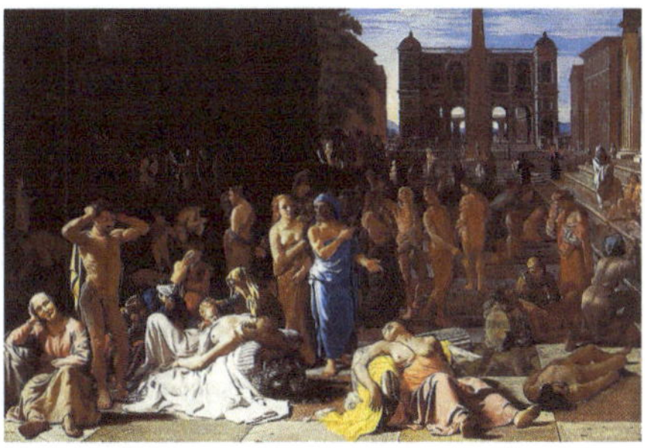

The image above is: Plague in an Ancient City - Michiel Sweerts.

In Plague in an Ancient City, the Flemish artist, Michiel Sweerts (1618-1664) is thought to depict here the plague of Athens in (430-427 BC) This vivid scene of devastation is not only haunting by the images of the dead and the dying but, perhaps, more poignantly of the anguish, crying, and sorrow of the living. Similar to COVID-19, the plague appeared suddenly, disappeared, and then reappeared again, leading to a deterioration of culture and society.

Like the present story, where George, our protagonist, returns from Afghanistan, the military roots of this picture is that the plague in democratic Athens deteriorated their army and led to their defeat by the militaristic Spartans. Was that a testimony to the fragility of democracy? Also allegorical to this story, George is haunted by nightmares of chaos, social disconnection, and suffering. This painting is a history lesson not only about the Athenian plague, the black death(1346-1353) or the Roman plague of the 1640's but also for our present times, where the theme repeats itself . The unfortunate dead are counted easily in a plague, but who is charting, in our present time, the aftermath of suffering, deterioration, and the rise in alcohol use as a consequence of trying to cope with the breakdown of societal norms?

Released by the Los Angeles County Museum of Art to be in the public domain

In early 2020, the world began to learn a new kind of fear: invisible, contagious, and everywhere. This story captures the first tremors of that era - and the ways a single phone call can awaken old dragons in the nervous system.

Uncertainty is a physiological stressor. The brain hates unanswered questions; it fills silence with worst-case scenarios. That is why sudden crises - war, illness, economic instability - often amplify substance use and relapse risk, even in people who have been stable for years.

Harrow's Field Note: Uncertainty as a Trigger

On a warm, clear night on March 5, 2020, John's cell phone

began to ring. He glanced at his watch and noticed that it was exactly 11.03 PM.

Who would be ringing at this time? he thought.

Four more rings, and John reached for the phone. Cellphones are like that - inevitable. John had enjoyed the time when letters came by mail rather than the imposition of an electronic device that was the norm now, which like a crying baby, was hard to ignore, and worse, difficult to resist. The calling code started with a +44, so he knew it was from England. Even more ominous! Surely the caller would have known the time difference, so it was either an emergency or a call to make a sad announcement. John often heard of the death of a relative or close friend in England late at night. That is usually when callers are able to get to him. After all, people died at all times, even in England.

Ring number 5!

John picked up the phone and said, “This is John; just tell me who died!”

There was a short pause at the other end, and then a chirpy voice answered.

“It’s Pamela, and as far as I know, everyone is fine over here. Even Astronuff.”

John breathed a sigh of relief and apologized for this curt answer.

After they exchanged pleasantries, John got down to asking Pamela what the matter was.

“Need some advice,” Pamela replied.

“Astronuff not available?” asked John.

“Well, he’s in sort of a funk. You know how he gets.

Chewing on his next brilliant idea to save the world. No time for me on this one. Far too clinical."

John was not sure whether to be flattered or annoyed, but he let the negative feeling pass. Not helpful to pursue anyway.

"Go on," he allowed.

Pamela started.

"Last week, I got a referral to see a curious young man. Let's call him George. He is 55 years of age. Several years ago, he had returned from the Afghanistan war with his regiment, the Royal Dragoon Guards, which, as you know, are a fierce lot. George had been deployed there with his regiment in 2010 and had done two tours of duty. He had not seen any action, and he mainly spent his time as an advisor to the local troops. Not one shot was fired by him or his mates at the barracks or at any time during the conflict. Once, there had been an air raid, but the enemy troops were worse shots than a bunch of gerbils with a peashooter. George had heard the loud explosions some miles away whilst he enjoyed some beers with his mates. He was never in any real danger.

"Having specialized in electronic communications left him feeling rather isolated from the rest of the men. Thereafter, he returned home to his wife, who, unfortunately, had decided to shack up with the local grocery delivery boy. George, however, reported that he was happy to be rid of such a faithless wife, as she had not really cared for him. In the last few weeks, he had come down with what seemed to be a mild cold and had taken to bed. Like the rest of us, he was asked to quarantine himself, even though none of his symptoms matched a diagnosis for COVID-19. All had gone well for the first week, as this was a great excuse to catch up on wartime movies.

George watched at least 2 nightly. His favorite was *Apocalypse Now*, and his favorite scene was the troop's beach-landing to the musical theme of the ride of the Valkyries. You know the one, from the beginning of the 3rd act of Richard Wagner's Die Walküre. He could recite almost every word. George said the scenes mostly amused him as he perceived real war, which he had not experienced, would be far more brutal. Indeed, he said his imagination of what that would be like was most horrifying.

"In between his movies, George watched all the news about the COVID-19 pandemic. He kept daily figures of the death rate and tried to imagine what it would be like to suffocate to death. Indeed, he had held his head underwater in his bathtub for as long as he could to try and simulate it. About one week ago, he heard that his ex-wife had caught COVID-19 and had died. George said that he had felt no sadness but instead had incorporated her dying, even though he had not been there, into his dreams. His dreams had become extremely vivid. George did not usually remember his dreams, but now he could not get images of men wearing World War II gas masks walking around different gravesites out of his head. The gravesites were always painted in bright colors, but more remarkable, they had surrealistic images of the people supposedly buried in them. It was as if the dead people had all painted their own faces on the graves, and then brutalized the very same images.

"George's dreams were a growing sea of faces, all of them staring back at him. He would try and contact these "dead people" by speaking to them, but when they opened their mouths, a string of airs always came out. At the most frightening part of the dream, he would hear distant explosions. George would awaken from his dream in a cold sweat and pace around the room. He had become obsessed with thinking that these dead people may be walking around him and was, therefore, always on his guard. About a couple of days before he came to see me, he had awoken so suddenly that he had fallen off the bed and banged his back badly against the bedside table, which had left him with a painful hobble to his gait, and made him experience some tingling down the side of this legs. George was wary that these people might seek to hurt him. During the day, he could hear his heart pounding, and each night when he switched on the television, he would feel his stomach churning, but somehow, he felt drawn to do so. George felt disconnected from his own body and fell into a cycle of despair. What he had not seemed to notice was that his delivery orders for Bombay Sapphire gin and tonic water from the local liquor shop had accelerated. George had chucked the empty gin bottles into various parts of the house that he was afraid of entering in case the "dead" were there, even though he knew they were a figment of his imagination. He refused to count exactly how much he drank, but he was now spending fifty pounds each day on booze and less than 5 pounds on food (mostly French fries). It occurred to him that a bottle of gin only costs about 20 pounds, and he knew his condition was getting out of hand, but did not know what to do about it. Last week, George had attempted to have a day of not drinking, but he could not cope with the urge to throw up every few minutes. He also felt intense heat all over his body. His hands now shook most of the time. On the day I saw him, he could barely remember who I was after every few minutes, and I had to keep repeating myself. The man had insisted that I wear latex gloves, not shake his hands, and to keep my face mask on as he did not want to get COVID-19, and the first question he asked me was where he could buy a ventilator without a prescription, and install it in his home. As George lived alone, he considered this would be a minor inconvenience once he could sort out the plumbing."

"Even more curious was how George had actually got to the clinic. The old lady who lived next door to him, also self-isolating from COVID-19, had knocked on his door to get a little milk. George had been so concerned about her fragile gait, the open wounds on her skin, and her foul-smelling clothes that he had thrown all caution to the wind. He had brought his elderly neighbor to our ER for medical help. It was as George walked into the accident and emergency department that an old friend of his, a former Dragoon, had noticed him hobbling and brought him swiftly to our walk-in neurological and neuropsychiatric clinic. Afterward, we took his history and conducted an MRI, which showed a mild injury to his lower lumbar spine."

Finally, Pamela stopped to take a breath. But before John could say anything, she threw in the hook, "Anything from that fancy American medicine you learned that could help this poor chap? And by the way, he hates taking medication so we cannot just start him on pills."

John was silent for a minute. This was quite the case.

"Let me sleep on it, and I'll call you in my morning after I've had a chance to mull over the impact of all these symptoms," he replied.

As John drafted this section during the first COVID winter,

sleep refused him. He listened to the rolling statistics—numbers that were meant to inform, yet often only inflamed the mind—and he noticed the truth beneath them: his own anxiety. Data can guide policy; it cannot, by itself, soothe the nervous system. That requires skills—breath, meaning, connection, and the deliberate re-training of attention.

Is everyone feeling like I do? John wondered.

The inventor of a 24-hour news channel was truly an evil genius! John had grown up with the news at 9 pm, and after that, you had to wait till the next day. Who had considered that millions of people would willingly agree to listen to so many tales of death, despair, and human cruelty all day long...and then turn it into an amusement?! We have all been numbed to the suffering of others, but now that it could be any one of us, at any time, the news had turned into a “stable” stressor. The perfect brain recipe for developing chronic stress! The same evil genius must have somehow figured out (but how could he or she have known?) that 80% of us have brains primed to receive good news. That is why most of us process bad news poorly, and it has to be repeated several times for us to get the true impact. Science and technology had been set to work against us in a true pandemic. It wasn’t that the health care services may or may not have been equipped to deal with the problem. Instead, it was worse. For now, we, as humans living in these times may not be fully equipped to deal with the deluge of personalized bad news - almost like having to attend one’s own burial every hour, on the hour.

John has a plan

At exactly 6:03 AM, John picked up his phone and dialed, and as soon as he heard the click of the phone, he spoke.

"Pamela, this is John! I know you did not call me late at night just for me to provide a diagnosis. Your genius plan was to see if I had been noticing what was happening all around me, and for that, I thank you. Calling so late at night was the symbolism to awake me from my mental slumber. Thank you!"

"Exactly six hours later, John!" Pamela exclaimed. "You do not miss a trick. You called me six hours after I called you. Six, the most harmonious of numbers and a symbol of peace." Peace be unto you this day John. What do you have for me about the case?"

John liked to be flattered by someone as smart as Pamela. He started to speak.

"As you know, although I like a diagnosis, I am much more into telling a story to understand the individual behind the disease. That way, it is easier for me to truly "see" him or her and come up with a plan that might work. George's problem started with his distant stress, which was when he was posted to Afghanistan. And that lay dormant for years. His wife leaving him was another stressor that got incorporated into his "stress matrix," and that became incorporated into his dreams. George's watching the war movies intensified the memory of his past stressors and linked that with his episodic memory. So, once the pandemic struck, and he was isolated, with fewer other materials to incorporate into his boring day, the new fearful memories evoked by COVID-19 became salient. His vivid dreams would qualify him for having a stress disorder, but I fear that its intensity is now so severe he has PTSD. And to make matters worse, he started to use alcohol to ease his constant state of anxiety and hypervigilance.

"Rather than give him a diagnosis of alcohol use disorder,

we can say his maladjusted drinking behavior is a problem. Both the chronic stress and excessive alcohol use that disturbed his sleep would have also inflamed his brain. His memory has begun to fail him as well, which underscores our conceptualization of his chronic stress. Additionally, the injury to his spine, whilst moderate, will require rehabilitation. George also seemed to be very much of a loner, so we need to find a way to help him feel "connected" whilst we are all still in isolation. He will need more treatment than just "pills," Pamela, if you wish him to get really better and have a fulfilling life. Let us remember too that his prominent complaint stems around his sleep problems."

Pamela listened quietly and seemed to be taking notes at the other end of the phone. She made a bullet list of John's recommendations. They were all orthodox treatments, but their application, and an initial attempt to avoid medicine, enabled a graded approach to wellness. Below is the graded response proposed by John to Pamela:

Dialectic Behavioral Therapy (DBT) and Cognitive Restructuring (CR)

Dialectic behavioral therapy is a targeted psychotherapy in which the therapist and client work together to develop personalized change-oriented therapies for wellness. This treatment would be particularly apt for George because it combines the elements of cognitive-behavioral therapy with emotional regulation and teaches how to cope with emotional stress. The particular element of CBT in DBT is cognitive restructuring. Here, emotional reasoning is strengthened, and distorted magical thinking is avoided. DBT has its roots in mindfulness training and interpersonal development, which would prepare George for other components of his regimen. DBT would also help in addressing George's developing alcohol use disorder. Because of the self-isolation of the COVID-19 situation, John recommended that these sessions start on alternate days using Zoom.

Hyperbaric Oxygen Treatment (HBOT)

Under normal partial pressures (approximately 95 mm Hg), a healthy individual would be expected to have a blood oxygen saturation of over 93%. Hyperbaric oxygen has primarily been used for the speedy healing of wounds and infections, due to the poor oxygenation of such tissues. Also, it has been used effectively for the treatment of traumatic brain injury, which can be exacerbated by hypoxia. This is because raising the fraction of oxygen from that in expired air from about 20% to almost 100% has a modest effect on oxygen saturation. Above atmospheric oxygen (i.e. > 1), ATA can have a marked effect on increasing oxygen saturation. HBOT has primarily been used in the treatment of PTSD arising from a traumatic brain injury with which there have been reported benefits.

The evidence for HBOT as a treatment for stress-induced dysregulation of fear is intriguing. Even though this study was done in animals, it showed that HBOT may decrease stress-induced high circulating levels of neurotransmitters and hormones activated during stress (i.e., norepinephrine and cortisone), and may, therefore, have a protective role in the brain.

HBOT is important as a reliever of the phenomenon of oxidative stress (discussed in detail earlier in this book), and his very recent spinal injury would benefit. Indeed, there is research that individuals who receive HBOT after an injury to their spine and become depressed or anxious may derive benefit from it. Even though much is not seen in an MRI of such an individual's brain, it does not rule out them having had even a mild traumatic brain injury, and HBOT would also be good for that.

The self-isolation during the COVID-19 crisis made John suggest that this be done with great care. Obviously, George would have to be brought to the treatment facility using a fully sanitized special vehicle every other day, and use the chamber specifically prepared for him (also fully sanitized).

Ozone Therapy

Ozone therapy was not recommended by John for George's treatment. Ozone therapy can be administered in various ways, but perhaps the most common method is autohemotherapy, whereby blood is withdrawn, exposed to the ozone, and reintroduced into the body. Evidence for the use of ozone therapy in medicine remains somewhat controversial, but there have been some stunning reports, although there are no formal controlled studies detailing its use in treating the respiratory symptoms in intubated patients with COVID-19. Decreasing ICU time and speeding up recovery would lessen the mental health impacts of the COVID-19 disease. These reports have come from China, Italy, and Spain; these countries being the ones that have seen the worst of the COVID-19 pandemic outside the USA.

Mindfulness and Meditation

To complement the DBT, John also suggested mindfulness training. This was an easy recommendation for Pamela to follow as she had also been taking mindfulness classes and guided meditation. These all will be done through video conferencing on Zoom. Even though it was being done remotely, everyone in the class could see each other, and it presented, at least for now, some sense of contact. This is very important in these types of cases since depression and thoughts of self-harm can occur suddenly without adequate monitoring.

Pills

John recommended that as soon as George became more comfortable taking some "pills", or if the earlier treatments were not fully effective, he would recommend a low dose of the medication topiramate. The author of this volume has described the use of topiramate for alcohol use disorder earlier in the book. Additionally, there is good evidence that topiramate (a Gamma Aminobutyric Acid agonist/Glutamate antagonist) could also be useful in the treatment of PTSD, and its actions could alleviate neuropathic pain and the effects of traumatic brain injuries (presumably by decreasing brain inflammation).

Exercise and Nutrition

John did not discuss exercise and nutrition with Pamela because he was aware she would run the necessary laboratory tests, as well as administer the supplements and vitamins needed to restore George's health. Pamela would also encourage aerobic exercises of at least 30 minutes each day, as it has been found useful in decreasing brain inflammation, improving mood, decreasing alcohol use, and enhancing memory.

Epilogue

This is a complex case on a new potential mental health issue, which may itself become a pandemic. Most individuals will be nowhere as complex as this, and will simply have anxiety and vivid dreams associated with the societal stress of watching the news or learning about COVID-19. There is, however, a pandemic brewing amongst those who have been admitted to the hospital, including the Intensive Care Unit (ICU), for the treatment of CO-VID-19. Those individuals will have a long path to recovery, with a high risk of major depression, anxiety disorder, alcohol and substance use disorder, PTSD, and Post ICU syndrome due to continuing medical problems. The approach to these simpler cases may be addressed by targeted psychological support. Presently, there is data that alcohol sales have increased during the COVID-19 pandemic, but it will take perhaps another year or two for all the mental health issues to be elucidated. John used all the information given to him to sew together a treatment plan for an unorthodox case using basic scientific principles. Such an application of basic scientific principles is needed to personalize a treatment approach that suits individual patients.

There is growing evidence that COVID-19 can affect smell, lead to confusion, and strokes. Brain damage caused by the COVID-19 virus is perhaps caused by the release of cytokines, which result in the inflammation of the brain. As the death rates from COVID-19 grow, so will the number of individuals with neuropsychological sequela.

An Introduction To The Science of Stress Awareness and Reactivity

Most of us are aware of the symptoms of acute stress or anxiety. Acute stress leads to the release of neurochemicals such as norepinephrine and epinephrine that stimulate and prepare the body for action. Typically, an individual would experience that their heart is beating faster, their mouth getting drier, "butterflies" building in the stomach, and that their senses of acuity and awareness are being raised. Increased blood pressure and oxygen delivery to the muscles also is typical. This can give rise to the fight or flight response, which prepares the individual to develop a response to the danger or stressful stimulus. Some individuals can develop panic attacks. These symptoms usually resolve within a short space of time, especially if there is no further exposure to the danger of stressful stimuli. In usual modern life, most of us can experience acute stress when asked to speak publicly or being "put on the spot" to perform some kind of activity. Sometimes, stressors are brief and naturalistic such as the separation from a partner or witnessing an accident.

If the stress or anxiety is chronic other symptoms can emerge. Individuals in a situation of chronic stress, which can be caused by isolation, develop a myriad of other complex symptoms. These can include a "crippling" level of anxiety such that the individual feels "paralyzed" or unable to respond to the stressor. Chronic stressors tend to be "stable" because the afflicted person does not know when the stressor will disappear. Chronic stress can cause a multitude of human diseases and can increase the risk of ulcers and chronic hypertension. Chronic stress can have a powerful effect on the immune system, especially on the white cells in the body called lymphocytes, such that the risk of infections is increased. Susceptibility to many cancers also may be driven by stress.

As seen in studies done in both humans and animals kept in captivity, this can lead to depression, such that the two, anxiety and depression, become part of the same condition. An important part of the human response that is typically disturbed in chronic stress is sleep. Importantly, there is a component of sleep called Rapid Eye Movement (REM) sleep in which individuals are physically unable to move but can have vivid dreams. Also, there may be difficulty initiating sleep, staying asleep, and another part of sleep, slow wave sleep (the most restful part of the sleep cycle), is also disturbed. Sleeping difficulties can exacerbate chronic stress, as the sleep abnormality alters the circadian rhythm of sleep, and the restorative effects of sleep are obtunded. The increase in cortisol and growth hormone in the morning to provoke normal physical activity, combined with the other disturbances of sleep, makes it that the person will usually complain of being "tired all the time."

In cases where there is an extreme or life-threatening danger or the perception of such danger, a post-traumatic stress disorder (PTSD), characterized by a state of hypervigilance, near-constant anxiety, and vivid, highly emotive dreaming can take place. The most common cause of PTSD is a recent sexual assault or threatened sexual assault. PTSD symptoms could have occurred in the past, such as sexual abuse in childhood, and in such cases, can manifest as distant stressors. PTSD can occur in wartime with exposure or threatened exposure to acutely dangerous situations.

Chronic stress can damage the brain. It seems to produce these effects by the exaggerated production of cortisol and the inhibition of neurons (brain cells), which communicate with each other to carry information. The seat of the fear response in humans is a structure called the amygdala (a pair of almond-shaped structures in the temporal lobe of the brain). Memories from another part of the brain called the hippocampus "talk" to the amygdala to condition the importance of the fear. In chronic stress, there is a reduction in the stem cells that produce neurons (brain cells) in the prefrontal cortex (the "thinking" area of the brain) that are vital for communication. Another peculiar change is that there appears to be higher production of another type of brain cell (oligodendrocytes), which causes a greater production of myelin (white matter) that sheaths the cell. Furthermore, there is strengthened connectivity between the hippocampus and the amygdala. In other words, when your amygdala is stimulating fear, it is amplified by the hippocampus (e.g., memories of all the bad things that can happen). Usually, this spiral or feed-forward fear process between the hippocampus and the amygdala is dampened by the prefrontal cortex (e.g., it says, "wait a minute, perhaps it is not so bad"). Without this dampening, the fear simply generates greater fear, initiating a vicious cycle.

The amygdala is worth an added mention. There is evidence of what is called hemispheric laterality, that is, one side of that structure in the brain processes a different function than the other. The right side of the amygdala may process negative emotions, whereas the left processes pleasant feelings. This is important because the right brain hemisphere is linked with declarative memory (facts that have to be "brought to mind"), and emotional memories of the event in time, place, and quality (i.e., context), which is called episodic memory. Thus, conditioning fear in the amygdala is associated strongly with evoking and coding deeper memories and associating them with the present episode. Fear is, therefore, a self-perpetuating phenomenon that can even be triggered by memory and can be self-sustaining once it had got started. Men and women differ in the development of their amygdalas. Whilst the amygdala is larger in men than women, it develops faster and reaches its maximum size earlier in women. The organ is also involved in the consolidation of long-term memory.

Some humans seem to be able to modulate the activity of their amygdala. As an example, Buddhist monks who practice a type of meditation based on kindness and benevolence seem to be able to modulate the amygdala, temporoparietal junction, and insula. Functional Magnetic Resonance Imaging studies (i.e., brain images that take pictures of how its specific parts are actually working, and to what intensity) show that expert meditators also seem able to have some control over their fear responses.

Damage to the amygdala can occur with repeated episodes of high alcohol consumption and withdrawal, and this may lead to a worsening of alcohol use disorder and, perhaps, opioid use disorder, by interfering with a brain protein called Protein Kinase C-epsilon.

Stress can lead to brain inflammation. Even more mundane stressors like a difficult working environment can induce alterations in the immune system such that it increases the production of microphages that can attack the brain. This phenomenon also has been associated with short-term memory loss.

Brain inflammation has been associated with the development of anxiety and depressive disorders.

Stress can kill you.

We have all likely heard the phrase 'stress can kill you', but much of that adage relates to the direct effects of stress on the heart. It may further be learned from an article by Dr. Ahmed Tawakol and colleagues published in the Lancet that stress activates a primitive part of the brain called the amygdala, to increase inflammation in the heart and the risk of heart disease. What is interesting is that there appears to be a feed-forward loop in which the more stress on the heart, the greater the activity in the amygdala, and correspondingly, even more stress on the heart.

For a brief recap, the amygdala is the part of the brain that mediates our strongest emotions such as hostility, violence, anger, and fear. Intriguingly, the amygdale may also process connections with deeper, perhaps even more negative memories that we might have had. If you like, it is part of the "dark side" of the brain. So, if your amygdala is over-worked, not only would you wish to flee any perceived dangerous situation, but your ability to perceive the amount of hostility you are encountering can also be distorted. Possibly worse still, the amygdala has connections with another part of the brain called the anterior cingulate, which tries to resolve fearful emotions. Think of the anterior cingulate as a boomerang that brings back all unresolved and uncomfortable memories and tries to sort them out. It is, therefore, reasonable to suggest that when this circuit between the amygdala and anterior cingulate is disrupted, there is an opportunity for emotions to be misread or misinterpreted. Thus, extreme fear can take us down a tunnel of even more fear. In other words, the "Frightened Brain" is more afraid than it needs to be or even should be! To paraphrase a famous saying by President Franklin D. Roosevelt: 'Fear fears fear itself!'

And, the frightened brain is not only bad for your mental health but can also damage your heart. While the research on the size of the amygdala and heart disease is interesting in itself, it is even more intriguing that another body of research shows that larger social networks might also increase the size of the amygdala. It would, therefore, be reasonable to propose that increased social behaviors and other interactions require the brain to negotiate how it will code a multitude of responses, from engagement to fear and anxiety. Since the amygdala is itself associated with the activity of other deep brain structures, as well as with the anterior cingulate, it is fair to say that we do all possess intricate networks that allow us to perceive, appreciate, and negotiate "dark" emotions. Furthermore, these effects of "dark" emotions in the brain can have an important effect on physical health, particularly on the heart. So, it would seem that a focus on creating and working to experience positive emotions, in addition to reducing stress, is an important way to staying physically healthy. Mindfulness through meditation can teach us to modulate powerful negative emotions. It would, therefore, seem fascinating to devote systematic and concerted study to the effects of various types of meditation or other mood training, as well as mindfulness on brain structure and function. To revert to what was mentioned earlier in this section, what is old, like meditation, may be part of a new wave that science might eventually prove to be important in improving both mental and physical well-being.

Elevate

Introduction to Treatment with Sex Hormones

In this short section, we will review the use and interactions between sexual hormonal treatments, well-being, and the use of alcohol. It's not uncommon for individuals with alcohol and substance use disorders to have complaints about sexual performance or suffer the consequences of aberrant sexual behaviors, such as developing infections (e.g., hepatitis) or sexually communicable diseases like HIV. Whilst some have advocated that excessive sexual drive should itself be classified as an "addiction", it is rarely clear what the deleterious effects of excessive sexual drive on the individual are, except in terms of social difficulties. Nevertheless, at present, simple behavior modification techniques are, perhaps, the most utilized to "normalize" sexual behavior.

Unfortunately, a discussion on paraphilias and highly deviant sexual behaviors are beyond the scope of this volume. But in this précis, the focus is placed on commonly used sexual hormonal treatments in men and women, and their interactions with alcohol.

Estrogen

Hormone Replacement Therapy (HRT) for women has been a mainstay of medical treatments for decades. There are hormone receptors all over the body, but the ones that have garnered the most interest are those involved in sexual functioning.

Since the 1940s, HRT has been available for the treatment of menopausal women who received estrogen to relieve symptoms such as hot flushes, night sweats, sleep disturbance, urinary frequency, and vaginal dryness. Estrogen has also been instrumental in the prevention of osteoporosis (i.e., bone fracturing). In the UK Million Women Study (MWS), although there were benefits to HRT, it raised some alarm to the fact that careful monitoring was still required, as there were risks of heart disease and breast cancer from the treatment. In addition, HRT has been associated with potentially significant health problems such as blood clots, gall bladder disease, stroke, and dementia.

To vastly minimize these risks, the lowest, most effective dose must be used. There is, however, also an issue of balance. Many of the women studied in large studies like the WHI study were older (in their mid-sixties) and often overweight. This population differs from women who, becoming menopausal in their mid-40's, wish to optimize their quality of life, but who still remain sexually active. Indeed, starting HRT within 10 years of menopause does not seem to be associated with an appreciably greater risk of heart disease. So, it is women over 60 who should generally not be started on HRT.

Hormones that are identical to those found in the body (bio-identical hormones) are being produced by pharmaceutical companies. The safety profile of bio-identical hormones and HRT appear to be similar. Some difficulties exist with monitoring bio-identical hormones, as they are not regulated by the Food and Drug Administration,

Once a woman eligible for HRT presents, and screening confirms suitability, the initial decision is whether to provide shorter or longer-term HRT. For instance, long cycle HRT can prevent periodic bleeding for up to 3 months and is preferable in women who use progesterone. Local estrogen creams can alternatively be used, but are less effective than systemically administered estrogen.

Menopause may be associated with mental health challenges. The most common are anxiety, depression, and stress reactions, although complaints of sexual dysfunction are also fairly typical.

Alcohol use disorder can complicate HRT and increase risks. Even the consumption of 2 standard drinks a day in women receiving HRT can increase the risk of breast cancer threefold, and rates, almost over five higher, have been reported in women who drink more than 2 standard drinks daily.

Prior to embarking on HRT, it is critical to get a complete physical examination, history, breast evaluation, and appropriate blood work from a family practitioner or obstetrician/gynecologist. If the therapy is given outside of these settings, there needs to be supporting information from the referring doctor.

It is advisable for women on HRT to avoid using alcohol as much as possible. If such women choose to continually drink, their checkup frequency should be increased, and the dose of HRT may require adjustment. Women on HRT may consult with a treatment center for alcohol use disorder to get help to decrease or stop their drinking. Furthermore, appropriate and personalized treatment needs to be chosen.

Testosterone

Testosterone is a hormone associated with increased sex drive, and in men, sperm production. Testosterone helps to build muscle mass and red cell production. It is present in both men and women.

Male testosterone levels decrease with age. The generally reported symptoms of this include low sex drive, erectile dysfunction, lack of energy, decrease in muscle mass, difficulty concentrating, body and facial hair loss, and importantly, mental health conditions such as depression, irritability, and a low sense of well-being.

Excessive alcohol consumption is associated with reducing testosterone production in the following ways:

a) It damages the Leydig cells in the testes that produce and secrete testosterone;

b) It uses a coenzyme called nicotinamide adenine dinucleotide (NAD+) for its metabolism, and this is the very same coenzyme used in testosterone synthesis;

c) It releases endorphins, which, although imparting a sense of pleasure, interfere with testosterone synthesis;

d) Increases levels of the stress hormone cortisol, which

decreases testosterone synthesis, and e) alcohol increases the conversion of testosterone to estrogen in the body.

Testosterone supplementation can be associated with a benign prostatic enlargement (hypertrophy), and an increased risk of prostatic cancer. It is, therefore, important to do a Prostate Specific Antigen (PSA) screening blood test prior to the administration of testosterone.

The hormone can be administered through various methods. Although it is possible to orally ingest testosterone, this is not the preferred route as the first-pass metabolism in the liver usually lowers how much testosterone is available in the blood. The more typical routes are transdermal skin patches and gels (e.g., *Androgel* and *Testim*) that can be applied on the skin where they are absorbed directly into the body. *Foresta*, *Axiron*, and *Androgel,* for instance, can be delivered by a pump, and *Natesto* is applied to the inside of the nose, and via c⊘ +injections and implants. Other means include injections that may be given into the muscles or implanted pellets (usually in the buttocks).

Typically, testosterone supplementation is not provided simply due to a low or marginal level of testosterone, but because the patient is symptomatic for the deficiency. Once testosterone supplementation has commenced, it is usually administered chronically because the exogenous testosterone suppresses the body's own ability to produce it. Thus, if there was a need to stop the supplementation, it would need to be undertaken gradually.

Low-dose testosterone may be prescribed to women who report a low sex drive, with no explainable causes, especially if they are menopausal. The long-term effects of providing women with testosterone are, however, not well understood. Prior to prescribing testosterone to a woman, it would be important to take a detailed psychosexual history, medical history, interview the partner, and search for stressors, anxiety, conflict, and mood disorders.

Summary

In healthy individuals, sexual libido, performance, and satisfaction is maintained and can be optimized by normative levels of sexual hormones. Alcohol can interfere with the levels of sex hormones in both men and women. Supplementation of sexual hormones in men and women should only be done pursuant to the provision of a full medical history and evaluation in individuals who are symptomatic due to measured deficiencies. Any supplementation should be done and monitored using accepted medical procedures.

As a special note, testosterone supplementation for women to boost sex drive is becoming more “vogue,” but this should only be done, and then with caution, following a very careful evaluation of the woman’s medical, personal, social, and psychosexual history.

A Better Way to Live

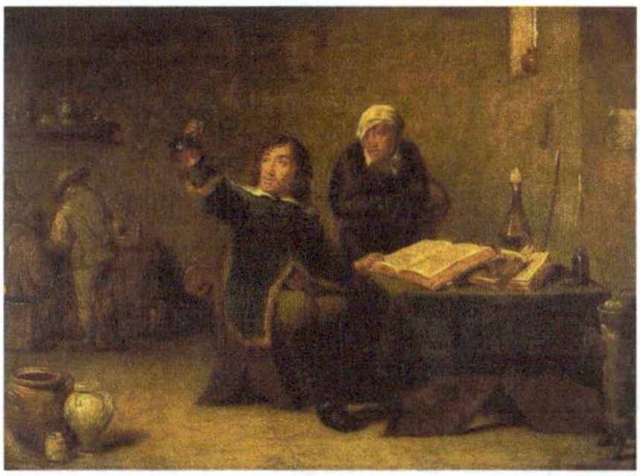

The image above is of a physician examining a urine flask that was painted by David Teniers II (1610-1690) (after) and is part of the Wellcome Collection. During his studies at Oxford University, Prof. Dr. Johnson was a Fellow of Wellcome, which granted him a research award to do his doctoral studies.

Any life can take a turn at the wrong junction.

Sometimes, these junctions are obvious and require conscious choices, but more often, simply going down a trail of decisions without correction hardens the path and makes a reversal impossible. Those that can see a path and make choices are really blessed because then, making an error of omission or commission lies in their hands, and the vicissitudes of fate are deleted from the equation.

John had casually picked up a magazine at a dentist's when he read about Morena. From the article, Morena was just the kind of professional woman every man would like to marry. She was a mind-blowing success of a record producer. Her mind was sharp, her wit cutting, and she had one of those contagious laughs that would brighten up any day. Her long reddish hair (presumably derived from her Celtic heritage) was always perfectly combed, and as such, was her signature. She definitely knew how to put herself together, and her charity work in Africa was legendary.

John read on.

Morena was married to a physician of no particular distinction; his only claim to fame being that he was married to her.

How did she pick such a fellow? John wondered.

He had always been intrigued to read the galling stories of female school teachers molesting their underage students, only to get to the mugshot and find out that these women were often beautiful, and on any given scale, would certainly have had their pick of a suitable man their own age. But insecurities can lie buried deep, at times for decades, until they surface as a chimera of the original injury. John knew well that no book could be judged by its cover - less so with humans - so why was there so much prejudice and pressure about how women were meant to look? He always thought this was all very sad, and a reflection of the primitive parts of the brain where strong emotions, but little reason, dwell.

Just when John turned the page and began reading about her tragic accident, he was snapped back into reality and found himself being ushered into the dentist's chair. He had always been suspicious of dentistry. A dentist who had practiced 30 years ago, perhaps further back, would still be familiar with a dental office now. The components were about the same; drills, chisels, cold water flushes, syringes with long needles, and more.

Why has nothing seemed to change?

John was terrified of dentists. As a child, his father would take him to his friend, who was a dentist. The man would numb John's mouth, and when the time came to do the actual dental work, the dentist would spend so long talking with his father that all the local anesthetic would have worn off. To curb his restlessness and obvious pain, the dental assistant would literally compress his chest with her weight so he could neither scream nor escape. On another occasion, she had switched on a set of traffic lights, obviously a gimmick to distract the patient, but since the sequence was the same, John had memorized it in under 2 minutes. He had soon learned, to his chagrin, that boredom makes the pain worse! This dental torture could last for an hour, and at the end of it, it was if he had been in a heavyweight fight, lost the fight, and would then have to watch the promoters, his father, and the dentist, arranging a rematch. Hadn't the boy suffered enough?

John's regular dentist was away that day, so he was assigned to a relief dentist. And who should walk into the room but Morena! Or so he thought.

Was it possible all that numbing gel made him hallucinate? How could that be? John soon came to his senses. What he was experiencing was a symptom called derealization. It can occur in situations of perceived significant stress as the mind starts to detach from reality. This had led to his misperception. Even John was not immune to neuropsychiatric symptoms, especially those invoked by stresses of the past not well buried!

"Good Morning John, my name is Victoria, and I will be looking after you today. Seems like you've had a good deal of work done," the stand-in said.

John gritted his teeth as if to form the last line of defense before she uttered those two terrifying words...

"Open wide."

John adjusted his glasses. This was not Morena and did not look anything like her. Victoria was a brunette (albeit with a reddish artificial tinge to her fragile-looking hair), and she was slightly overweight. What was most striking about Victoria was her pale skin and unusual walk, which resembled a hobble. Her eyes looked tired and sleepy, and her voice sounded a bit hoarse. John gave her a smile, and just as he was lowered into the chair, and the bright lights were turned on, he wandered into a trance. For the first time in a dentist's chair, time seemed to pass away quite quickly. However, as the room flooded with classical music, and the drilling stopped, he knew she was taking another restroom break. John was astonished that Victoria had turned out to be the gentlest of souls and had done all she could to make him comfortable. It had worked too. He could trust her!

John thought nothing of that encounter with Victoria until

an early Tuesday morning in March. It was one of those days when dewdrops collect on the leaves of flowers, and the hum of insects signaled the beginning of Spring. John loved Spring. He had always been told by his friends from Africa that dewdrops were tears of joy from the angels and that drinking the early morning dew brought new life. John performed his Spring ritual of drinking some of the dew from the leaves in his garden and had headed off to work only a few miles away.

For a Tuesday morning, the clinic was quite busy. Out of the corner of his eye, he caught the sight of someone sitting in the waiting room. John never liked to see anyone waiting; the clinic's policy was no one should have to wait more than eight minutes. Any longer, and there would be no charge! Before John could utter a word, his assistant, John, caught his eye and mumbled, "There's a lady named Victoria here waiting to see you. She doesn't have an appointment. What would you like me to do?"

"No worries, John, I know her," John replied. "She's my dentist, perhaps the best in the business. Now, it's our turn to look after her."

John knew what that meant: 'we're going well beyond our own limits of beyond for this patient.' If she wasn't happy, maybe she would.... The consequences just didn't bear thinking of! John showed Victoria into John's office, and she seemed quite tired.

"Hello, John, surprised to see me? I have heard so much about you. I thought I'd give you a try. Let me cut to the chase - I'm tired all the time. My own doctor called it burnout and prescribed anti-depressants, which just made me feel worse.

Also, I had a total hysterectomy last year, and I'm on the pill at my age! Shortly after this, my husband left because he found sex with me unsatisfactory. He said he was too old to fiddle with all the gels we have to use, and that I always looked bored anyway. I really loved him and wished he did not leave, but then he met a much younger girl, and from then on, he was no longer mine. Do you think you can prescribe something else?"

Victoria began to cry, and John handed her the white handkerchief from the left breast pocket of his suit, then waited until she regained her composure. He began:

"I'm so sad to learn what had happened to you. It all must have been terribly painful, and with your busy job, it must sometimes feel have felt lonely, and as though there was no way out. We do things differently over here and take it one step at a time to get to the bottom of the problem. We try to investigate the problem first rather than push pills or any treatment. It's going to be a long day."

John ran the usual genetic, blood, and urine tests on Victoria and noticed that she had glucose in her urine and low phosphate. But none of this was dangerously low. Her estrogen level was low, which would account for her thinning hair and lowered libido, but he had a nagging feeling that something was being missed. John went into Victoria's side room to tell her that she needed better control of her estrogen supplementation, which was easy to fix, but again, she was in the restroom, and the pitcher of water was empty.

Like a lightning bolt, it struck John. How could he have not put all the symptoms together? The empty pitcher of water, the lazy eye, the fatigue, thinning hair, cancer treatment, and a hobbled gait. It all led to one possibility, but he needed to see Victoria to be sure. As Victoria entered and sat on the examination bed, John asked, "May I please look into the back of your eye?"

Et Voila! There it was, she did have ptosis (a lazy eye), but more importantly, her optic disks (the visual part of her eyes) were curved. John glanced again at the lab results and noticed that her thyroid-stimulating hormone levels were high (which would give her the hyperthyroid symptoms that included the hoarse voice, rapidly beating heart and fatigue), and she was leaking proteins from her kidneys.

"I think I know what you have Victoria and can now help you, but first, I want to do one last thing," the doctor explained.

John knew he had to figure out why she had a hobbled gait. As happenstance would have it, the doctor who had been renting the space prior to John's practice had left a bone density machine in the corner of one of the rooms, as it was too heavy to move and the clinic doors were too small. John whipped out his cell phone and placed a call.

"John, you are the most technical person amongst us. Do you think you can get that bone density machine working?"

"Depends. If it's a software thing, no problem. If it's hardware, not a chance."

John's practice was full of over-qualified people, and his assistant had been at the top of his class in computer technology at the world's second-best university (and we all know where that is). John jumped to the task, and in 15 minutes, Victoria's bone density scan had begun. John was restless and read the results of the scan as soon as they started popping up. Her bones were full of holes, a condition called osteomalacia. She had been hobbling, with what is known as an antalgic gait, to take pressure and pain off her joints.

John came back into Victoria's room excitedly.

"I am now certain that I can help you! You have a rare condition called Fanconi syndrome. All your doctors missed this diagnosis because they were all focused on your hysterectomy but ignored that you had so many other symptoms. Additionally, Fanconi syndrome is usually a disease of children, because, at that age, it is usually genetic. It is much easier to spot in children because they stop growing. You acquired the disease, not because of your genetics (we checked) but because you must have received a medicine called cisplatin during your cancer treatment. I am not a metabolic specialist, but Dr. Jeffrey, who works with us, is a card-carrying endocrinologist and can help with all our hormone treatments. I will introduce you to him. One more thing, you can stop the anti-depressants. Instead, I would like you to meet Barbara, our psychologist. She will help with your loss. I shall, like for everyone, stay on top of all your treatments. As you know, one way or another, we will be seeing each other every month, and I certainly don't want you mad at me or falling asleep with a drill in your hand."

Victoria was overwhelmed but managed to give a wry smile at his joke and thanked John.

Dr. Jeffries worked with Victoria for about one year until he was fully satisfied that he had her estrogen replacement under control (which restored her enjoyment of sexual relations), monitored and restored her dehydration with selective fluids, provided phosphate (about 2g per day) to correct the imbalance, corrected a complicated problem of too much acid in the blood (called metabolic acidosis) by giving an alkali (bicarbonate), and of course, vitamin D infusions to improve bone density and structure.

Barbara, the psychotherapist, engaged in a mixture of cognitive-behavioral therapy (CBT) to curb her depressive symptoms, while assertiveness training was meant to prevent burnout and taught her to deal with disappointment. Eventually, she did reunite with her ex-husband, but that was not a happy ever after tale, as he soon returned to his paramour. But, by that time, Victoria had gained the strength to be a woman in her own right! (*A woman in your own right* by Anne Dickinson 1982).

Victoria had taken that fork in the road and found a better way to live. Her next relationship seemed much happier. She recounted that not only was this achieved through Barbara's good works but from a book she had recommended that had taught her how to have those difficult conversations and keep a kind, loving, and harmonious relationship going (*Difficult conversations and what to say in tricky situations by Anne Dickinson, 2006*).

John never finished reading Morena's story, nor did he care to. The metaphor was obvious, two poles, Morena and Victoria juxtaposed; two choices, yet only one true solution.

Being surrounded by harmony, love, and friendship is not only a better way to live but the only and best way!

Dying for Kilimanjaro

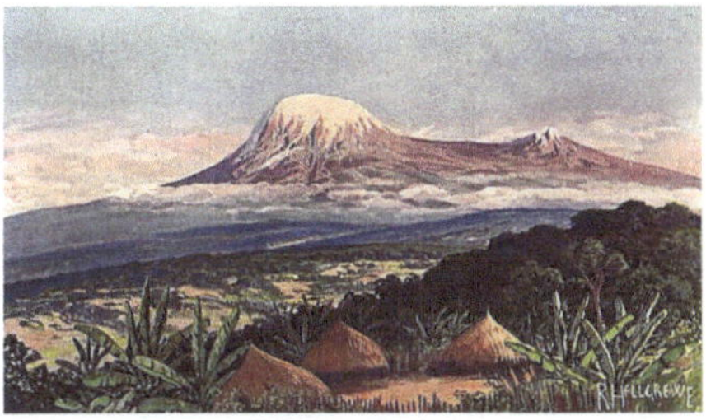

The image above is: Mount Kilimanjaro (5,885 m / 19,340 ft), a dormant volcano in Tanzania with three cones - "Kibo", "Mawenzi", and "Shira" - painted by Rudolf Hellgrewe (1860-1935).

It had been a long day at the clinic for John, and he was looking forward to getting home and simply watching re-runs of *Star Trek*; with its resounding message of hope for humanity. But then, a middle-aged, distinguished-looking African gentleman knocked on the practice door. John glanced at his watch - it was already 6.30 pm. Who could it possibly be?

John let the gentleman in. He recognized the man immediately, and as he let in his trouping entourage, wondered why an appointment had not been made. Reaching out to greet the gentleman, who we will call Nelson, John noticed two important things which, unknown to him at the time, would be of critical importance in what was to transpire. First, there was the fact that despite his considerable wealth, his hands were rough as if he had been working in the fields all his life. Next, the doctor took note of a scar or birthmark on his lower lip, which was only evident when he smiled.

Nelson was incredibly formal, which complemented his outfit. He wore a crisp blue Saville Row suit, white wing collar shirt, 7-fold hand-woven silk tie with a Stefano Rici emblem, and most striking of all, shoes from A Diciannoveventitre, distinguished by their natural worn look, which the casual observer would simply think looked dirty. John knew that this was not going to be an easy encounter, and it was getting late. He recognized Nelson from an amusing story he had read about the man in a newspaper. Despite his considerable wealth and education, Nelson was highly superstitious and was known for his preference of herbal remedies and mixing herbs, which John now knew he must have picked for himself. Having graduated from 2 Ivy League American universities, both with doctoral degrees in the sciences, Nelson returned to his home in Tanzania to build a fortune in the sale of rare metals through several untraceable subsidiaries. But that was not his claim to infamy.

Allegedly, Nelson had gone to a traditional doctor (what

some would call a "witch doctor") to purchase a bulletproof jacket. Reportedly, the witch doctor had asked for a sum many times higher (some say it was over a million dollars in cash) than the usual Kevlar-based bulletproof jacket, to produce one for him made of woven silk. The silk jacket was described as having beautiful red embroidery with purple tones on the lapel, and a picture of Mount Kilimanjaro hand-stitched on the right breast pocket. This seems to symbolize strength and purpose. When Nelson visited the traditional healer to collect his bulletproof suit, he had insisted on testing it. At first, the traditional healer had protested but eventually agreed to try it out on a member of Nelson's entourage. Allegedly, a gun fired at the hand of Nelson's entourage member by the traditional healer, pierced right through leaving an ugly bleeding wound. The traditional healer had protested that the suit had been made specifically for Nelson, linked to his very own spirit and not that of his entourage member, and would surely have worked for him. The healer blatantly refused to try on the jacket and have the gun fired at him. Reluctantly, the intended user had put the healer-made jacket on, and as the traditional healer had fired, Nelson had turned his face to see him fleeing out of the corner of his eye. That sudden action, which saved Nelson's life, had produced the glancing wound of the bullet on his left lower lip, which was evident when he was not concealing his smile. The traditional healer was never again found, despite an extensive national search. How could someone as smart as Nelson fall victim to such a trickster?

It was Nelson who broke the ice.

"My good doctor, I read about you in a magazine on the way here and just had to come in and see you. I am staying at the Four Seasons, so it was no effort at all to just come down and check if you were open."

"Pleased to meet you," John answered, while Nelson and his entourage swept behind him to take up seats in the lounge. "Perhaps you would prefer some privacy?" John asked.

When he had ushered Nelson into a private room, the man began to speak.

"That story everyone has read about me in the papers is not true. I actually got this wound from my wife, who got angry after finding out I had cheated on her. But I had to preserve my dignity, so I conspired with the press to make up that tall tale. No one of my intelligence would ever do a thing like that. But instead of people being amused, they actually believed it."

John was unusually perturbed and anxious. He wondered whether anything that Nelson would say to him had an iota of truth. Worse still was the fact that the man had the resources to ruin John if he got things wrong. He knew he had to tread very carefully and disguise his obvious unease.

John eventually spoke up.

"Yes, Nelson. People will believe anything. Some even believe the world is flat and that tectonic plates are coming back together to form one world. More still find it is hard to grasp that Earth's magnetic north pole is moving towards Russia, and consider it a CIA conspiracy theory."

"Are you ridiculing me?" the guest fired back.

"Not at all, the world and its beliefs are not always centered around logic, but rather a perception, and sometimes, that perception is nothing more than the person telling a story. You probably remember that news clip of the

Iraq Minister of Information telling the world to believe him despite the very American tanks he reported to be many miles away in flames with their occupants rolling behind him."

At this, Nelson roared with laughter.

"I enjoyed that too! What was the name of the guy again? Oh, I remember now; Mohammed Saeed Al-Sahaf. It should really have been Al-Sa-DAFT! The man was robbed of getting an Oscar."

Realizing that he had now broken the ice with Nelson, John decided to proceed with the interview.

"How can I help you feel better about yourself?" he asked.

Nelson was now quite relaxed and started telling his story as he stroked the thin, white, and patchy hair on his head.

"Well, it all began a few months ago. I was having trouble with my old lady. She is always at my throat and insists on always getting not just the last word, but the only one. It usually feels like I'm going deaf with her screaming in my ear, and I have to leave home. Then when I do, she accuses me of seeing a mistress. I did try to have something once but could not even complete the task because I could not get it up. I was so ashamed that I started to drink. But that only made it worse. My desire was sky-high, but my performance with the missus was terrible. At first, I put it down to the conflict I was feeling then, but I could not even get visually aroused. It was then that I did visit a herbal healer who brought me some dried fruit from a flowering tree that he claimed to have encountered at the foothills of Mount Kilimanjaro. These I grew, and now cultivate in my own garden. It's a pretty strange looking tree, and I add the dried fruit and some honey into my beer. I like the drink so much as it gives my savory beer a sweet taste. And it also seemed to wake me up down there. All seemed to be well until I began to get a pain in my chest every time I drank my favorite concoction. Now, I am left with the problem down there, and I am afraid that I cannot drink my favorite beer with my dried fruits anymore."

John asked some follow-up questions:

"How much do you drink? Has controlling your drinking ever been a problem for you, and if so, when? Have you ever felt guilty about your drinking or had to have an eye-opener in the morning to function? Have you ever tried to quit drinking and couldn't? Have you had any symptoms or bodily sensations if you try and cut down on your drinking?"

"That's easy," Nelson replied. "I have about 2 or three beers every other day with my herbs, 2 doubles of Oban Little Bay (a single malt scotch whiskey) and do not drink on Sundays. And no to all the other questions."

John was always impressed by people who had a love of single malt Scotch whiskey, though the people he knew with such tendencies were prone to either obsessive behavior or peculiarity, above all, had great taste. In his experience, single malt liquor drinkers spent so much time around the ceremony of preparing their drinks with frozen rocks and just the right amount of water that they did not usually binge drink. But, naturally, there were many exceptions to this soft unscientific impression.

John swiveled his chair around so as to face Nelson more directly.

"I will need to take blood tests, perform a thorough physical examination, and send you for an MRI of your heart and head. The results of the blood tests will be available tomorrow afternoon, and we shall have the MRI results about an hour after they have been done. I am glad you brought some of your herbs with you, which we will test as well, although that might take a little more time. In addition, I would like you to spend an hour or so with our psychologists, and a few other technicians to complete your history. So, by tomorrow our team should have a response on how best to help you. For now, try and enjoy your stay here, and I will see you same time tomorrow."

As Nelson got up to leave, he stared at something in the corner of the room and seemed transfixed.

"Oh. The twins?" John said, noticing his guest staring. "They were given to me by a very special friend named Bruce, who runs an antiquities store in Miami that you might like to visit. Like you, he seems to have an eye and fascination for the exotic. Indeed, these were special twins. Bruce did not know the history well when he gave them to me, but I was happy to fill him in.

"The Yoruba believe that when a child is born, one half of the soul is left in heaven. With twins, the connection to the spirit world is doubled, and the bond is inseparable. This bond is so strong that if one of the twins dies, the spirit moves into the second twin. So, to prevent the other twin from suffering the same fate, the figure is provided for the spirit to move into. The carved figures are always identical, even for non-identical twins, to symbolize the unity between them. In the Yoruba language, this is called ère ìbeji. In that incarnation, the dead twin lives and is commemorated. Twins are sacred in Yoruba culture, and a source of good luck and fortune. And now, a fact I doubt many people know; the rate of twins born in West Africa is four-times that in the rest of the world, and no one knows why that is.

"Perhaps, the Yoruba are simply an extremely lucky group of people. If you are superstitious and you get a hold of these twin carvings, do not separate them, because that would be bad luck. That is why they are kept on a pedestal in the corner, all by themselves, where no one can disturb them. Remember, legend says that together they are a source of goodwill and beneficence for all who enter."

At that point, the eyes of the two men met, and they exchanged a knowing nod.

The Next Encounter

John was looking forward to seeing Nelson again, though he knew he had been in the clinic for a couple of hours, completing his evaluations. But first, there was a brief team meeting to get to. Of course, John had seen the MRI results and blood tests. He had also managed to identify, strangely, the herb Nelson had been taking! The doctor was hopeful that the solution would please Nelson.

It was 6:45 pm when the team regrouped to brief Nelson about his condition and the various treatment options (which they would design specifically for him) that were available. On this occasion, John had decided it would be best if he led the meeting.

"Good evening, Nelson. Let's start with the really good news: The MRI of your heart and head reveal no significant damage, and you are in relatively good health but quite overweight, though I shall return to that. Your lab results, with an out-of-range high level of acetone, would make many clinicians run a large number of tests and label you prediabetic. But, in reality, you are less than 10% over the upper boundary of normal, and I believe that our nutritionist sitting over there will help you to get things under control. We will, of course, keep a watchful eye over it as a precaution."

John went on.

"Next, I want to address your excessive alcohol consumption. You are drinking well above the safety limit - in fact, about double of that. NIAAA guidelines basically state that men who drink more than 4 standard drinks in a day (or more than 14 per week) and women who drink more than 3 in a day (or more than 7 per week) are at increased risk for alcohol-related problems. I have done quite a good deal of research on this myself and would say that despite your excessive alcohol use, you would not currently meet the criteria for an alcohol use disorder. Also, your lack of family history would suggest that we may be able to manage this with a brief intervention and some education. For that, Barbara, our psychologist whom you have been speaking with, shall meet with you, even by videoconferencing, two to three times a week. She will also ask you to keep a diary recording your daily drinking habits, which should be easy as you will be doing something similar with the nutritionist. We know that you would not agree to give up drinking alcohol, so let's work to develop personal drinking goals for you within that safe limit. If that does not work, we will provide you with a medication called nalmefene, which you will take before you start drinking to help you curb the drive. I doubt that will be necessary in your case, but at least we are thinking and planning ahead".

John was now smirking and looked pleased with himself.

"Now, for the genie in the bottle. I am no botanist, but I was able to look up the shape of the leaves and the description of your symptoms. Also, I reached out to an old friend this morning, who is a botanist in Kenya. We are certain that the flowering plant you have been putting in your beer is called *Kigelia Africana*, from the genus Bignoniaceae I knew this was it because you told me you were taught not to eat the fresh fruit since it is poisonous. Instead, you were to dry the fruit and then mix it with your beer, bee pollen, and honey to produce your drink. You have learned that if you let it ferment a bit, your beer would actually taste stronger and richer, and I suppose you have grown used to this peculiar fermented broth. And yes, it does have some aphrodisiac properties, but you probably only got that effect by tasting a bit of the unripe fresh fruit, which is a no-no and comes at the expense of putting a strain on your heart as it contains alkaloids. It also can cause a stroke. *Kigelia Africana* in the right hands is an amazing medicine for many ailments, including rheumatism and ulcers. Traditional women have also learned that rubbing the sap into their breasts makes them firmer."

John paused for a short intake of air before blurting out the final statement.

"And now for the diagnostic prize. That abrasion on your lower lip had nothing to do with the alleged bullet wound or your wife. They are blisters caused by chewing into the fruit produced by *Kigelia Africana*."

Even for this experienced team, this piece of medical detective work was indeed special!

Recovering his composure, the doctor became more serious.

"The thinning hair, even at your age, was a tell-tale sign considering your ethnicity. As I suspected, you do have a low testosterone level. In fact, it is half of what it should be. Your prostate is in good shape, so help is at hand if you agree to let us inject you with testosterone pellets. It will take about 4 weeks to reach peak effect, and this will have to be monitored every month to ensure you are within normal limits. The only catch to this, I must warn you of, is that once started on them, it really can be lifelong, as your own body's ability to make testosterone gets suppressed. Would that be all right with you?"

Nelson nodded and smiled in appreciation.

"We are not quite done yet," said John, adjusting his seat to rest beside Nelson's.

"We really need to help you fix your relationship with your wife; if you both wish it. Too much conflict is stressful and will certainly not help you with getting aroused or having a loving relationship. Trouble is, you have to find the right therapist for both of you. With the wrong therapist, it will result in disaster. Some of those quacks out there focus so much on having sex that they forget that it's not about performance but intimacy. You need to learn your wife's love language, and for that, there is a most excellent lay book. But to guide you on this path, Barbara has offered, if you wish, to call your wife and help work out the best therapist for you two. It might happen, of course, that you both choose Barbara, but that has to be your choice."

Nelson seemed grateful, and as he left the clinic in Miami that day, he seemed to have had a weight lifted off his shoulders.

Epilogue

Nelson continued to get better.

Indeed, when John called him up a few months later, he seemed to be beaming.

"Doctor, as I was leaving your practice in Miami, I got myself a few bottles of that love potion of yours, Ignite, and it seems to have helped along with the testosterone injections to keep me in the right zone. My wife enjoys it and whatever it does too. We usually "take things slow," mixing it with just one shot of tequila for the evening. In fact, that's my only drink of the week except for the odd Scotch now and then. Old habits are hard to fight. Barbara has been just brilliant, and she stayed with us and brought in Roger, who is also on your team to guide us through our marital hurdles. My wife and I felt like we each had our champions, but they always seemed to find a compromise.

"We have learned so much from them. And as for that flowering tree, I thought it best to cut it down. Just too much temptation, and my imagination kept running wild..."

At that point, John thought it prudent to steer the conversation on to the safer ground.

"You really should visit Mount Kilimanjaro," he exclaimed. "It's not too far away from you, and there are safe day trips and people to meet and chat with. It's the great outdoors, and there is just no sky anywhere that is like the African sky".

Both men laughed, bid their goodbyes, and hung up the phones.

* * *

Signature Reflection: Dying for Kilimanjaro

A late-day knock at the clinic door becomes a reminder that healing is not only the absence of symptoms - it is the return of wonder. John Horacio Harrow hears, beneath the practical question, a human invitation: step outside the tight radius of worry and remember the sky.

If you remember one thing: recovery expands when your world expands.

- The dragon's disguise: exhaustion that convinces you you've "earned" collapse.
- The turning point: a simple human connection that redirects the nervous system toward hope.
- A practice to try: schedule one small "Kilimanjaro" each week - something outdoors, embodied, and bigger than your screen.

Clinical lens: novelty, movement, daylight, and social connection are not "extras." They are biology - inputs that regulate stress chemistry, sleep architecture, and cravings.

Chapter 13

Some Concluding Remarks To Book 3 Of 3

You've reached the end of Book 3 - the closing volume of this Signature Series, and the beginning of what comes next.

This book thrusts you into a world in upheaval: pandemic fear, social unrest, and the quiet loneliness that can make any mind feel unsteady.

By now, one truth should feel clear: brain disorders are also disorders of experience. The brain and mind are inseparable - biology and story braided together.

You've also seen the paradox of the brain as a "silent organ": we depend on it for everything, yet rarely give it deliberate care until something breaks.

And you've watched John return to Africa - the cradle of his youth - to meet old fears with new tools, and to discover that courage is not the absence of pain, but the decision to move through it.

Et futurum exspectat! - The future awaits.

Chapter 14

Concluding Remarks To The Series

This is a continuing story - because brain wellness is not a finish line. It is a practice, a relationship, and a way of living.

At the heart of this series are composite stories designed to bring complex ideas down to human scale - so that neuroscience becomes not just information, but insight.

Brain optimization, cognitive resilience, and the prevention of decline are real medical priorities - and also deeply personal ones.

Few of us wake up thinking, “How do I care for my brain today?” Yet our attention, our moods, our relationships, and our choices all depend on it.

Health systems often reward treatment more than prevention. But prevention is where freedom lives - because it gives us options before crisis takes them away.

Overindulgence in alcohol, drugs, food, and sex can be understood not as moral failure, but as brain-based patterns - patterns that can be interrupted, re-trained, and healed.

It is striking how many treatment centers still operate without the full benefit of modern, evidence-based addiction science.

Sometimes the barrier is not malice, but inertia: tradition, limited training, limited resources, and the mistaken belief that "experience" alone is enough.

But the science is here. The question is whether we will use it - with humility, rigor, and compassion.

In the Six Rings series, Professor Dr. Bankole Johnson has attempted to weave individualized treatments into narrative - so the reader can feel the method, not just read it.

Some characters share aspects of The Professor; others are entirely their own. Together they reflect a central idea: growth is possible, but it requires honesty.

As you read, notice the emotional development across the volumes. Knowledge expands - but so does empathy, discernment, and the courage to change.

There will always be critics. That is not a problem. The point of the series is not to win arguments, but to widen understanding - and to invite better care.

Six Rings strives toward a vision of healthcare at its best: where resources are used wisely, practitioners are well-trained, and treatment respects the whole person.

It is a hopeful vision - maybe even utopian at times. But the direction matters: towards what is true, what is helpful, and what heals.

Life is not perfect. Healthcare is not perfect. Neither are we. Still, we can keep moving - one honest step at a time.

The journey continues.

Chapter 15

Further Reading and References

Johnson BA, Roache JD, eds. *Drug addiction and its treatment: nexus of neuroscience and behavior*. Philadelphia, PA: Lippincott-Raven Publishers; 1997.

Johnson BA, Ruiz P, Galanter M, eds. *Handbook of clinical alcoholism treatment*. Baltimore: Lippincott Williams & Wilkins; 2003.

Johnson BA, ed. *Addiction medicine: science and practice*. New York: Springer Science+Business Media; 2010.

Johnson BA, Roache JD, Javors MA, DiClemente CC, Cloninger CR, Prihoda TJ, Bordnick PS, Ait-Daoud N, Hensler J. Ondansetron for reduction of drinking among biologically predisposed alcoholic patients: a randomized controlled trial. *JAMA*. 2000;284:963-971.

Johnson BA, Ait-Daoud N, Bowden CL, DiClemente CC, Roache JD, Lawson K, Javors MA, Ma JZ. Oral topiramate for treatment of alcohol dependence: a randomized controlled trial. *Lancet*. 2003;361:1677-1685.

Johnson BA, Rosenthal N, Capece JA, Wiegand F, Mao L, Beyers K, McKay A, Ait-Daoud N, Anton RF, Ciraulo DA, Kranzler HR, Mann K, O'Malley SS, Swift RM, Topiramate for Alcoholism Advisory Board, Topiramate for Alcoholism Study Group. Topiramate for treating alcohol dependence: a randomized controlled trial. *JAMA*. 2007;298:1641-1651.

Anton RF, O'Malley SS, Ciraulo DA, Cisler RA, Couper D, Donovan DM, Gastfriend DR, Hosking JD, Johnson BA, LoCastro JS, Longabaugh R, Mason BJ, Mattson ME, Miller WR, Pettinati HM, Randall CL, Swift R, Weiss RD, Williams LD, Zweben A, COMBINE Study Research Group. Combined pharmacotherapies and behavioral interventions for alcohol dependence - The COMBINE Study: a randomized controlled trial. *JAMA*. 2006;295:2003-2017.

Johnson BA, Ait-Daoud N, Seneviratne C, Roache JD, Javors MA, Wang X-Q, Liu L, Penberthy JK, DiClemente CC, Li MD. Pharmacogenetic approach at the serotonin transporter gene as a method of reducing the severity of alcohol drinking. *Am J Psychiatry*. 2011;168:265-275.

Johnson, BA. Addiction Medicine. Published by Elsevier, 2019

Chapter 16

Signature Edition Epilogue: When Dragons Lose

When dragons kill, they do it quietly, one small permission at a time: a rationalization, a shortcut, a secret. A single night that feels survivable, then repeats until it becomes a life.

And the inverse is also true. When dragons lose, they lose quietly too: one honest moment at a time. One decision, too small for applause, strong enough to change a trajectory.

Across these three volumes you have met the dragon in many disguises: high-functioning success; grief; anxiety; loneliness; trauma; ambition; boredom; pain; and the seductive myth that numbness is a form of rest. You have also seen the cost: the narrowing of a life, the thinning of relationships, the erosion of self-trust, and the way the brain can mistake relief for healing.

Clinical credibility matters here because hope deserves evidence. The brain is plastic. Reward pathways can be retrained. Stress systems can be calmed. Sleep can return. Meaning can be rebuilt. Recovery is not a single epiphany; it is a learning process - neural, behavioral, relational - repeated until it becomes familiar.

That is the purpose of the Six Rings. Not a slogan. Not a moral lecture. A scaffold: a way of holding a person steady long enough for biology to stabilize, for the mind to soften, and for choices to widen again.

Preparedness is the courage to look directly at what is happening, without collapse and without denial. It is the moment you stop negotiating with the dragon and start gathering resources: support, structure, and truthful information.

Restoration is the body's long exhale. It is hydration, nutrition, sleep, movement, and the repair of neglected rhythms. It is the recognition that the brain cannot do its best work when the body is under-supplied.

Evaluative Personalization is humility with a microscope. It says: one person's pathway is not another's. The right intervention depends on history, biology, co-occurring conditions, and the real world that waits outside the clinic door. This is where science becomes compassionate precision.

Awareness is the skill of noticing the dragon early. Reactivity is the skill of responding with intention instead of reflex. Elevate is the skill of building a life that is more compelling than the craving, one that makes sobriety feel less like deprivation and more like return.

If you remember only one thing, let it be this: you are not the worst moment of your life. You are not the most painful craving you have ever had. You are not the relapse, the lie, the lost years, or the shame. Those are events. You are the person who can learn from them.

The dragon loses when the story changes: from "I can't" to "I can try," from "I'm broken" to "I'm rebuilding," from "I'm alone" to "I'm supported." It loses when secrecy becomes speech, when chaos becomes routine, and when suffering becomes data instead of destiny.

May this Signature Series be a companion in that change. And if you are reading this for someone you love: thank you. Your steadiness matters more than you know. Compassion is not weakness; it is an evidence-based intervention.

The next chapter is not written for you; it is written by you, one ring, one day, one breath at a time.

- **Withdrawal** — Physical and psychological symptoms that occur when a substance is reduced or stopped after dependence; severity varies and can be dangerous with alcohol.
- **Trigger** — An internal or external cue (emotion, place, conflict, fatigue) that increases the probability of craving or use.
- **Toxicology** — The study of substances and their effects on the body; in medicine and forensics, toxicology helps interpret impairment, exposure, and risk.
- **Tolerance** — Needing more of a substance to achieve the same effect, reflecting adaptive changes in brain and body.
- **Stigma** — Social devaluation or discrimination that

can delay care and worsen outcomes; reducing stigma is itself a therapeutic intervention.

- **Shame** — A painful belief that one is fundamentally flawed; shame fuels secrecy, and secrecy fuels relapse risk.
- **Reward pathway** — Brain networks (including mesolimbic circuits) that learn what is “worth pursuing.” Substances can hijack these circuits.
- **Resilience** — The capacity to adapt and recover after stress or adversity; resilience is trainable and supported by biology, relationships, and meaning.
- **Recovery** — A process of sustained improvement in health, function, and quality of life. For many, recovery includes but is not limited to abstinence.
- **PREPARE / Six Rings** — A whole-person framework: Preparedness, Restoration, Evaluative Personalization, Awareness, Reactivity, Elevate.
- **Precision medicine** — An approach that tailors prevention and treatment to the individual—considering biology, environment, behavior, and context.
- **Opioid Use Disorder (OUD)** — A medical diagnosis defined by impaired control over opioids, craving, tolerance/withdrawal, and continued use despite harm.
- **Neuroplasticity** — The brain’s ability to change with experience; recovery leverages plasticity through repetition, environment, support, and physiology.

- **Motivational interviewing (MI)** — A counseling method that helps people resolve ambivalence and strengthen intrinsic motivation for change without confrontation.
- **Mindfulness** — Training attention and awareness in the present moment with less judgment—often used to reduce stress reactivity and strengthen self-regulation.
- **Lapse vs. relapse** — A lapse is a brief return to use; a relapse is a sustained return. Clinically, both are treated as data—signals to adjust support and strategy.
- **HPA axis** — The hypothalamic-pituitary-adrenal system that regulates stress hormones; chronic dysregulation can worsen mood, sleep, and craving.
- **Harm reduction** — Strategies that reduce risk and damage even when abstinence is not yet achievable (e.g., safer use practices, overdose prevention).
- **Forensic science** — The application of scientific methods to questions of law and investigation (e.g., toxicology, injury interpretation, timeline reconstruction).
- **Executive function** — Higher-order brain skills—planning, inhibition, working memory, flexibility—often strained by stress, sleep loss, and addiction.
- **Dopamine** — A neurotransmitter central to reward prediction, motivation, and learning; dysregulated dopamine signaling can intensify craving and habit formation.

- **Cue reactivity** — The brain's learned response to triggers (places, people, emotions) that predict use —often experienced as automatic craving.
- **Craving** — An intense urge or drive to use a substance, shaped by cues, stress, memory, and expectation of relief or reward.
- **Comorbidity** — The presence of two or more conditions at the same time (e.g., AUD with depression, anxiety, PTSD, or chronic pain).
- **Clinical credibility** — The commitment to evidence-based claims, accurate mechanisms, and appropriate uncertainty—so hope is anchored in truth.
- **Chain of custody** — A forensic principle: the documented handling of evidence from collection to analysis to court, protecting integrity and credibility.
- **Brain wellness** — An evidence-informed approach to optimizing brain function across sleep, nutrition, stress regulation, relationships, purpose, and medical care.
- **Biomarker** — A measurable biological indicator (e.g., lab value, imaging signal, physiologic measure) that can inform risk, diagnosis, or treatment response.
- **Allostatic load** — The cumulative "wear and tear" on the body from repeated stress and dysregulated adaptation.
- **Allostasis** — The brain and body's process of

achieving stability through change—adapting to stressors over time, sometimes at a biological cost.

- **Alcohol Use Disorder (AUD)** — A medical diagnosis defined by impaired control over alcohol use, craving, tolerance/withdrawal, and continued use despite consequences, on a severity spectrum.
- **Addiction** — A chronic, relapsing condition in which compulsive substance use persists despite harm, driven by changes in reward, stress, learning, and executive control circuits.

This glossary is provided for educational clarity. It is not a diagnostic tool or a substitute for professional medical advice. Terms are simplified for readability while keeping clinical meaning intact.

Glossary of Key Terms

Chapter 17

Reader's Companion: The Six Rings Toolkit

This companion section is designed to help you translate story into practice. It is educational - not a substitute for professional care - but it can help you organize what you already know and identify what you may need next.

If you are in immediate danger, experiencing withdrawal, or feel unsafe, seek urgent professional help. The bravest move is often the simplest one: ask for support.

1) The Dragon Check-In

Use these prompts as a private, judgment-free snapshot. Answer honestly. If several items are "often" or "almost always," consider bringing this page to a clinician, sponsor, counselor, or trusted support person.

1. I use alcohol or substances to change my mood more than to enjoy a moment.
2. I hide, minimize, or rationalize my use - especially to people who care about me.
3. I feel relief when I know I can access the substance (even before I use it).
4. My sleep is disrupted, and I rely on substances to fall asleep or to wake up.
5. Stress or conflict triggers a strong urge to numb, escape, or "shut off."
6. I tell myself "this is the last time," then repeat the pattern.

7. My use is affecting my health, relationships, work, or self-respect.

8. I feel anxious or irritable when I try to cut back, even for a short time.

9. I have stopped activities I once loved - or I do them less - because of use.

10. I feel stuck between shame and craving, as if there is no clean way forward.

2) A One-Page Six Rings Map

Choose one small action from each ring. Small is not weak; small is repeatable. Repeatable becomes reliable.

Preparedness

- Name the pattern in one sentence (no excuses, no self-attack).
- Tell one safe person the truth.

Restoration

- Prioritize sleep protection (consistent wake time, dim lights, no late stimulants).
- Hydrate and eat protein early in the day.

Evaluative Personalization

- List your top 3 triggers and the top 3 consequences you fear most.
- Discuss evidence-based options with a professional (therapy, medication, group support).

Awareness

- Practice a 60-second body scan when cravings arise.
- Notice the first cue (time, place, person, emotion) rather than the last.

Reactivity

- Delay: commit to 10 minutes before acting on an urge.
- Disrupt: change environment immediately (walk, shower, call, step outside).

Elevate

- Schedule one meaningful activity weekly (service, art, sport, learning).
- Repair one relationship through a single honest conversation.

3) The "If-Then" Plan

Write your own sentence stems and keep them visible. The brain loves rehearsal - use it for your advantage.

- If I feel overwhelmed after work, then I will ______ for 15 minutes before I decide anything.
- If I feel the urge to isolate, then I will text/call ______ and tell them one true sentence.
- If I slip, then I will treat it as data, not a verdict, and I will do ______ within 24 hours.
- If I am ashamed, then I will remember: shame grows in secrecy; healing grows in disclosure.

Chapter 18

Signature Discussion Questions

These prompts are written for personal reflection, clinical training discussion, and book-club conversation. Use what helps; skip what doesn't.

1. Where did you see the dragon disguised as something "reasonable" or "normal"? What made it hard to name?

2. Which moment in the stories felt most psychologically true - and why?

3. How did stress, sleep, and social context interact with craving in the characters' lives?

4. What did compassion look like as an intervention (not just a feeling)?

5. Which ring - Preparedness, Restoration, Evaluative Personalization, Awareness, Reactivity, Elevate - felt most underdeveloped for the characters? For you?

6. How did secrecy and shame amplify the problem? What reduced them?

7. Where did the clinical science strengthen the emotional truth of the narrative (or vice versa)?

8. What was the turning point that wasn't dramatic - but mattered?

9. How would you describe the difference between relief and healing in your own words?

About the Author

Prof. Dr. Bankole Johnson DSc., MD., MBChB., MPhil, DFAPA, FACFEI, FRCPsych, DABDA, DAASCP is an award-winning physician-scientist, neuroscientist, and molecular geneticist, whose work bridges brain wellness, addiction medicine, practical realities of clinical care, and forensic medicine.

Across research, teaching, and clinical leadership, he has focused on evidence-based approaches that reduce suffering, restore function, and treat addiction as the medical disease it is—without moralizing, and without abandoning the human story behind the data.

He is the creator of the Six Rings / PREPARE framework—an integrated model that brings together assessment, personalization, restoration, and long-term brain optimization. The approach, and the philosophies behind it, form a cornerstone for the future Privée Clinics ecosystem.

In parallel with his clinical work, Prof. Dr. Johnson has contributed to the scientific literature on the neurobiology and treatment of addictive disorders, including the development and evaluation of pharmacologic strategies and precision-minded approaches.

This Signature Edition is published by THE INSTITUTE OF REGENERATIVE MEDICINE (www.irmnfoundation.org/home).

www.ingramcontent.com/pod-product-compliance
Lightning Source LLC
LaVergne TN
LVHW051127210926
848482LV00001B/3
* 9 7 9 8 9 9 4 5 9 1 2 4 6 *